# HEALING AT HOME

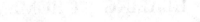

# HEALING AT HOME

## A Guide to Health Care
## for Children

Mary Howell, M.D., Ph.D.

BEACON PRESS · BOSTON

This book is dedicated to the memory of Child Health Station, written with affectionate regard for Donna, Judy, and Ellen, and presented in honor of our children: Eli, Allison, Aaron, Eve, Sarah, Peter, Christine, Sam, Diane, John, Jeff, Daryl, and Nick.

May we all continue to become healthy, in reality as well as in reminiscence!

"Pulse Rates in Infants and Children" (chart 15) and "Respiratory Rates in Infants and Children" (chart 16) from *Textbook of Pediatrics*, 9th edition, by Nelson, Vaughan and McKay. Reprinted with the permission of author and W. B. Saunders.

"Normal Blood Pressure" (chart 17) from *Pediatric Cardiology*, 3rd edition, by Nadas and Fyler. Reprinted with the permission of author and W. B. Saunders.

Information for charts 1–14 have been adapted by Carol Rose from Growth Charts put out by the Department of Health, Education and Welfare.

Library of Congress Cataloging in Publication Data

Howell, Mary C
   Healing at home.
   Bibliography: p.
   Includes index.
   1. Children — Diseases.  2. Children — Care and hygiene.  I. Title.
[DNLM:   1. Child care — Popular works.   2. Pediatrics — Popular works.   WS113.3 H859h]
RJ61.H85      618.9′2005      77-88329
ISBN 0-8070-2368-X

# CONTENTS

# CHARTS

# ACKNOWLEDGMENTS

I send thanks to all those medical professionals — technicians, doctors, and nurses — who have shared knowledge and skills with me. To the many mothers who have shared with me their own wisdom and experience I send respect, gratitude, and special fond greetings. Finally to Joanne Wyckoff and MaryAnn Lash, editors at Beacon Press: your unfailing grace makes the struggle of our process a pleasure, even apart from the product.

# FOREWORD

We ordinarily think of *healing* as repair. The bias of our present medical system has led us to consider healing as no more than restoration from an illness or injury back to a previous state of being not-ill or not-injured. We also talk about healing as something that one person does to another.

This book has a somewhat different focus. The root of the word healing means whole, sound, healthy. Healing can thus be understood to be a continuous and ever-changing process: a reach for a state of vigorous and blooming good health. Healing is a continual transformation *toward* healthiness.

As a continuous process, healing goes on every moment of our lives. This corresponds, of course, to what we know about our bodies: in every instant, from birth onward, all of our tissues and organs are in a state of flux, with molecules moving in and out, proteins breaking down and being freshly constructed, functional mechanisms becoming more or less efficient. This continuous transformation can be in a direction of greater healthiness, or in a direction of lesser health. But we are never static.

Healing, then, is much more than the repair of specific disease states. At the end of an episode of illness or injury we may be healthier, stronger, and more vigorous than we were before, or we may be weakened, damaged, and less healthy. But we are never just the same as we were before. Healing, in this sense, is a process of transformation that goes on *within* each person. Others can assist us in our healing, and we can provide that assistance to others in turn. But each individual body contains the potential and the capability for self-healing. We heal ourselves.

When we think about healing, then, we are reminded that we heal ourselves from within. In a broader sense, *Healing at Home* is about the assistance that mothers provide to children as children learn to heal themselves.

Groups like NAPSAC (The National Association of Parents and Professionals for Safe Alternatives in Childbirth), the American Public Health Association, the Women's Health Network, and the Feminist Women's Health Centers have recently made great progress in providing responsible and reliable information about self-help home care for adults. However, there has been relatively little of this sort of information directed to mothers to help them in the care of children. Mothers have been left without the information or understanding necessary for wise and skillful home health care.

I am a pediatrician and a child psychologist. I have known many mothers, have helped them take care of their children, and have talked with them about their own lives. I have seen their collective ingenuity and competence in bringing their children through an astounding variety of illnesses and injuries. I have also seen their uncertainty, their lack of a sense of pride and self-confidence in the care of their children, and their habitual stance of apology to the professionals they consult. I remember — with a pang of identification for myself and other mothers I have known — a young mother who brought her firstborn son, one month old, to my office. She was exhausted from nights of waking to feed him, and like most mothers of firstborns had many questions and worries about his healthiness and the appropriateness of her care. He was beautiful, and I told her so. She said, "I know," and burst into tears. I put my hand on her shoulder and asked her what was wrong. She said, "I know he's beautiful — he's perfect. And I'm so afraid I'm going to ruin him."

Much has been written about mothering by professionals, medical and otherwise. But very little of this so-called wisdom has been written by mothers. As Adrienne Rich argued in *Of*

*Woman Born*, this has led to the construction of an *institution* of mothering that differs from the actual *experience* of mothering.

I am convinced that any useful information presented to mothers about healing at home must begin with an understanding and recognition of what it is like to be a mother in this society, to act as agent for one's child in relation to medical experts, and to carry out the responsibility of caring for one's children when they are ill or injured. This understanding and recognition must focus simultaneously on mothering competence, and on the basic lack of support that medical professionals traditionally give to mothers.

I know, from years of working with mothers, the wide range of skills and thoughtful knowledge they can and do exercise in caring for their sick children. For any illness or injury that is cared for at home, mothers do what needs to be done. I have known mothers to give elaborately skillful care to children with long-term and medically complex problems. I have known mothers to react with speed, good judgment, and great skill in emergencies. And, of course, mothers deal every day with pains and hurts that are considered insignificant by medical professionals but, cumulatively, have profound significance for children's healthiness and for their capacity for self-healing. These instances range from the day-to-day decisions about the foods that are offered, to the immediate care of small wounds, scrapes, and bumps, to the sophisticated process of deciding when a child is too ill to go to school.

Mothers sometimes make mistakes as they try to assist their children in healing. Sometimes they do too much, or too little; sometimes they fail to notice signs and symptoms that signify more serious disease and a need for professional consultation. But I am convinced that for most mothers, most of the time, these mistakes are made only because it is so very difficult to learn the information and skills that are needed for home health care for children. The mistakes are not made because mothers are stupid, or because they are not concerned about their children's welfare.

Medical professionals who give care to children are not trained to respect mothers as agents for their children. In fact, there is much in medical training that allows the medical expert to see himself or herself as someone who rescues children from the incompetence of their mothers' care. I have found this attitude in textbooks and journals written for medical professionals. I have witnessed encounters between mothers and medical professionals that make this attitude clear. And I have been told, by mothers, of countless instances in which doctors, nurses, or other medical experts made the mothers feel incompetent and stupid.

Those who are trained in the various professions of medical skill have come to believe that the knowledge and skills they have learned are to be jealously guarded, not to be shared with layfolk. There is an economic basis for this point of view — medical experts earn money for knowing what layfolk do not know. There is also a psychological basis, for there is power, self-aggrandizement, and security in belonging to an elite group that is allowed to hoard its knowledge and skills.

In fact, most of the information and understanding that mothers need to provide really skillful and competent care for ill and injured children at home could be easily taught, and easily learned by mothers. But the combined attitudes of mothers and medical experts in relation to each other have made this teaching and learning not only rare but difficult.

In an earlier book (*Helping Ourselves,* Beacon Press, 1975) I asserted that those who were privileged to have professional training had a responsibility to share what they know with layfolk. This book is part of my sharing, part of my fulfillment of that responsibility. When my own children are sick or injured I usually care for them at home. Some of what I have learned from my professional training is very useful in home health care. I have also learned a great deal from other mothers in the course of my medical practice, things that I was never taught in my professional training. I mean to share with you as much as I can of what I have learned — through my training and experience — about assisting children in their healing at home.

Over and above the *reparative* healing, the overcoming of illness and injury, there is the much larger topic of healing as a continuous reach for healthiness, the transforming process that goes on every moment of our lives. Medical experts do not know a great deal about healthiness, or about this kind of healing. But as mothers — as the single most constant and effective influence in the lives of our children — we also transmit to them our attitudes and beliefs about this broader kind of healing. If medical professionals cannot inform us about this, perhaps we mothers can reconstruct what our foremothers knew, can examine what we know from our own lives, and can invent guidelines for helping our children. When I talk about healing as a continually transforming process toward healthiness, I am sharing with you what I and other mothers of my acquaintance have pondered over and puzzled through. My concept of this sort of healing is itself a process, for I am still struggling to learn even as I teach what seems to be a useful beginning.

Not long ago, when I was working in the wards of a big city hospital, I was strolling through a corridor in an adult section of the hospital. A middle-aged nurse was wheeling a very old woman out of her room, and she bent over the wheelchair to say, "Haven't you heard of that? Well then, let me teach you." I thought then, that must be one of the most truly beautiful sentences in our language: *Let me teach you.*

Learning how to teach each other, and valuing that effort, might be a key to the kind of human community in which we and our children could regain a sense of health. Learning how to learn, with openness and skepticism mixed, might allow us to go forward in our tenuous groping for, and understanding of, the healing process. The skepticism is as appropriate for what we are told by our mothers (who know some "old wives' tales" about sickness and health in children) as for what we are told by medical experts (who know some "old docs' tales"). This book is written with a large dose of that skepticism, and should be read in that spirit. It is about learning to learn, and learning in turn to teach.

Fathers and mothers alike should read and learn about the skills for home health care. However, mothers still provide the major share of child care and to these mothers I have addressed my book.

The book is directed to the mothers of children from birth through adolescence. It is of particular use for children between the ages of 6 months and 12 years. Tiny babies express dis-ease* in subtle ways; mothers will want to consult professionals frequently when interpreting and remedying the disease of a young infant. As a child grows through adolescence, s/he will increasingly take responsibility for his/her own health — having learned from the mother for the past many years how to understand dis-ease, to ask for help from professionals, and to strive for health.

The book urges frequent consultation with medical professionals. These may be doctors, but other experts can be equally helpful and sometimes are more accessible: nurses, nurse-practitioners, physicians' assistants, midwives, and various technicians.

The first chapter sets a stage. The mind cannot learn unless it is ready to learn. Many of our prevailing attitudes about medical experts, disease, and healing cripple our abilities for healing at home. We must start with a fresh look at professionalism, healing, and health.

The second chapter proposes an overview of healthiness, and a way of looking at strengths as well as dis-ease. We will then consider how to assess a child's momentary state of healthiness, beginning with the kind of information that we have by knowing the child very well, knowing his/her past history of strengths and dis-ease, and living with the child on a moment-to-moment basis. The organization of this information — which corresponds to a medical "history" — is always the point of beginning in an assessment of health. The information

* By its Middle English origins the word "disease" means simply "a lack of ease." In the professionalization of human affliction, we have given the term "disease" the connotation of medical diagnosis. We tend to assume that the only *real* diseases are those for which doctors have labels and some clear understanding of cause and cure. The form "dis-ease" is used throughout the book to remind us that we must consider, as we think about health, any and all conditions that give "a lack of ease." The form "disease" is also used, but only in cases that refer to specific disease states.

is *subjective* in the sense that it reflects the child's own experience, reinforced and elaborated by your experience of knowing her as her mother.

The third chapter outlines the steps of an examination of the child, another kind of information-gathering. This information is *objective* because it is gathered by your eyes, ears, hands, and perhaps even smell and taste. What you learn from an examination is information of the moment, but to be useful it must reflect back upon what you know about the child from previous examinations. You will know, when you listen to a child's breathing with a stethoscope, that an episode of dis-ease has brought a change because you have listened before and you know what the breathing usually sounds like. Much of this objective information that you assemble to think about, like the subjective information that you began with, is only an elaboration of what you already know. So much of our mothering — looking, grooming, holding, and caressing — brings us information about the child's body; we only need a framework for coordinating and thinking about mothering in a manner that will direct us to assist the child in healing.

The fourth chapter considers the kinds of remedies that are available for us to use at home, from the drugs that are available only on a doctor's prescription, to herbal remedies, to specific skills of care. It suggests ways to think about what the child might need to heal an instance of dis-ease.

The fifth chapter gives a number of examples of symptoms and signs of dis-ease that can be cared for at home. In each instance, the subjective information and the objective information that must be thought about and searched for are indicated. Sometimes there are additional perspectives that you will want to consider, including questions that you might raise in consultation with a professional. Finally, remedies are suggested for each particular illness or injury.

The next chapter offers some guidelines for thinking about the healthiness that we want our children to strive for in their daily living. It focuses on nutrition, exercise, and relaxation.

The seventh chapter points to the difference between safeguarding the care of your child in an episode of dis-ease for which you have sought professional consultation, and the efforts that you can make to change the medical-care system so that professionals are more responsive to the needs of mothers and their children. In each case your tactics and strategies will be quite different, and it is important that you reserve your efforts to change the system until a time when your child is not under professional care.

In every instance, this book gives examples. This is by no means a compendium of everything you need or want to know about child health care. The intent instead is to suggest ways for you to think about health and dis-ease, about the assembling of subjective and objective information, about the choice and use of remedies, and about controlling your relationships with medical experts. I respect your wisdom, and the intensity of your caring about your children, enough to know that with a framework for thinking about healing at home you will apply. your own ingenuity and competence to any specific instance.

The book is not a polemic against the use of professional consultation. My urging instead is that you know what information you want from medical experts, that you use any visit to a professional as an opportunity to ask questions and to learn, and that you gain a clear sense of what medical experts can and cannot do for your child.

The most important ingredient that you bring to your assistance to your child's self-healing is your intimate knowledge of that child. In this you have information that no medical professional can match. The information and skills that you can learn for healing at home are, for the most part, fairly simple to use. This is a well-kept secret of the experts. But your store of information about your child is unique and irreplaceable. Your child's trust in you is an invaluable ingredient in healing assistance. And your ability to teach your child about healthiness and healing — from your intense desire that your child be well — is one of the most precious gifts of your mothering.

# CHAPTER 1

# Thinking About Health
# and Dis-Ease

Before we can begin to think about the ways that mothers can
help their children to heal themselves, we must examine current and powerful attitudes about health and dis-ease. We need
to consider the prevailing notions about repair and restoration
from illness and injury that are taught us by medical experts.
We must look carefully at the habitual relationships between
medical professionals and layfolk. And we must think about
a new concept of health.

Our attitudes about these matters are well entrenched.
These attitudes are consonant with a social philosophy that
controls much of our behavior by the simultaneous promise of
perfectibility — the notion that if we did what we ought to do,
what professionals and experts tell us to do, our lives could be
free of pain and affliction — and the motivating forces of guilt
and blame, which warn us that if we or our loved ones suffer
any pain or affliction it may be our fault. The promise of
perfectibility and the press of guilt and blame make us turn
increasingly to professionals for advice, to deny our own competence and understanding, and to become helpless suppli-
cants for direction in every aspect of our lives.

Mothers are caught in these attitudes like everyone else.
But for mothers, there is the added dimension of *responsibility*
for the welfare of children. If we find it difficult to make de-

cisions about our own lives, based on thoughtful self-knowledge but contrary to the wisdom of professionals, it is infinitely
more difficult to feel confident about the independent decisions we make about the lives of our children. "First, ask an
expert" can become a guiding principle, a way of safeguarding
ourselves against the accusation, from others or from ourselves,
that we did not do as well by our children as we might or
should have done.

## How Medical Professionals Think About Health and Dis-Ease

Medical professionals do not, in fact, think about health very
much at all. The focus of all medical training is on specific
illnesses and injuries. Health is defined primarily as a negative
state — the absence of specific illnesses and injuries. For instance, a blood test that does not show a specific illness is
called a "negative" test. Medical experts argue that their job is
to overcome disease, pain, affliction, and even death. In fact,
the driving energies in the work of the medical profession are
invested in a kind of contest against illness and affliction;
death is the ultimate enemy. Many doctors feel that they have
lost a battle, have been defeated, when a patient dies.

This sense of contest means that, for most doctors, their
interest is always focused on the detection and cure of specific
disease states. A healthy person is of little interest to most
doctors. The work that brings them satisfaction is the clever
discovery of an interesting "case" and the application of skillful (and often technologically elaborate) remedies. Many of
these remedies that doctors now use, especially those that are
applied in hospitals, have some real risks of harm to the patient. These risks of harm can, of course, be justified when the
disease seems more harmful if left untreated. This kind of
heroic medical practice is what doctors, nurses, and hospitals
now do best.

Of course, many of our complaints and worries about our
health are not diagnosable as specific disease states. Many
more cannot be cured by specific remedies. Contemporary
medical science can explain only a small proportion of our

ills, and has curative remedies for an even smaller proportion of those. In the care of children, doctors trained in pediatrics often grumble about how rarely they see interesting cases. They are trained to be clever detectives, and to apply heroic remedies. Most children, however, are basically healthy — although perhaps not as healthy as they might be — and most of their complaints do not warrant risky remedies. In fact, most of their episodes of dis-ease are quite well cared for by their mothers at home.

*Dis-ease* is not the same as *the diseases* that doctors are interested in discovering and curing. The word dis-ease reminds us that healthiness is a goal, perhaps seldom reached. To strive for healthiness means that we must take notice of all of the small instances of distress, dysfunction, disability, and disfigurement in our attempts to reach a state of greater serenity and vigor. Many instances of dis-ease are of importance to health and of concern to mothers in the care of children, but often they cannot be classified with official diagnostic labels and have no precise and curative remedies.

Doctors want to believe that medical science will, in the near or even distant future, overcome all suffering and affliction. That hope for perfectibility sometimes forces doctors to dismiss real but undiagnosable dis-ease as trivial, or even to deny that it exists. The child who stumbles when s/he runs may not have an orthopedic problem that can be labeled or treated, but s/he has a kind of dis-ease and the mother wants to help her child. The child with a passion for sweet foods has another kind of dis-ease; so does the child with dry skin that feels itchy and tight. Mothers are sometimes told that their concerns about these and similar matters are not legitimate; sometimes it sounds as if doctors and nurses deny that the dis-ease exists.

Similarly, medical experts tend to know little about the kinds of remedies that mothers have traditionally used for their children at home. Sometimes they are disparaging, stating that peppermint tea or a rub with a liniment "does nothing" to help a child. As we shall see, there are more kinds of remedies that just those that cure.

Because medical professionals have been trained to think mostly about curative remedies, they tend to think of themselves as healers. Although they may give lip service to the patient's own healing potential, they would like to think of themselves as the agents of cure. Only when a patient does not respond as expected do we hear about the patient's healing potential — and then hear that the patient was run-down, or a smoker, or poorly nourished, and thus unable to benefit from the remedy that was expected to cure.

In fact, the blaming of patients for their own illnesses has become quite popular among medical professionals. As layfolk ask why, with so much money going into medical care, we are not feeling better and living longer, medical experts have taken to blaming the victim. It is argued that the way we live makes us sick. Often little notice is taken of such factors as poverty, the kinds of foods available to us to buy, the stresses of our work and schools and marriages, and the chemical pollution of our air and water.

Blaming the victim in the context of medical care for children usually means blaming the mother. Mothers are scolded, openly or subtly, for worrying too much about their children's health and bothering the doctor unnecessarily; for bringing an ill child to be examined before the illness has reached the point where a certain diagnosis can be made; for waiting too long to seek professional consultation, so that the illness is more difficult to treat; and for applying home remedies on the strength of their own judgment and experience. Many pediatricians say, "I enjoy taking care of children, but oh, those mothers." Some nurses who work with children adopt this same attitude. Other nurses (and some doctors), especially those who are mothers themselves, have a greater and more sympathetic understanding of the mother's role as agent for her child's health care.

## Relationships between Medical Professionals and Layfolk

If doctors, nurses, and other medical technologists are committed to winning in a contest against pain, disability, and

death, it is easy to see why they o
about dis-ease that cannot be labeled
to understand why all affliction is lo
to be overcome or ignored, something
into one's life.

In fact, if we look on healthiness ε
after, then all dis-ease and affliction ha\
even argue that the experience of afflicti
manness of existence. Unless we know w          to feel
pain, how can we know how to take care     others in pain?
Many mothers would agree that it is the affliction (not dis-ease) of pregnancy and childbirth that gives them the first impetus to empathize with the distress of their helpless and wordless infants. This empathy is the base upon which all mothering care is constructed.

More significantly for mothers, if all dis-ease is either avoidable or curable, then we are perplexed and saddened by the manifest suffering of our children. Most of their complaints and disorders fall between blooming good health and the diagnosable and curable diseases that doctors know about. There are scraped knees and cut lips, diarrheas and coughs, twisted ankles ard headaches that must be attended to. We usually get little or no help in these concerns from medical experts.

At the same time, we are increasingly tied to the seeking of professional advice. A system of threats cautions us that only doctors can discover those lurking and disabling, if not life-threatening, conditions that might be signaled by diarrhea or a headache. As medical science gets more and more technologically complex, and as more and more rare but dangerous diseases are identified and named, it is easy to dread that "there might be something seriously wrong."

This sense of dread applies equally to adult and child. The difference is that children are in the care of their mothers, and mothers are held responsible for the welfare of their children. This means that it is even easier for mothers than for other adults to take on an attitude of supplicant seeking for professional advice and the guarantee that all is well.

The most difficult and most perplexing block between

perts and layfolk occurs around the notion of the ...ing that comes from within, and the concept of health- ...s as the goal of healing. The child is doubly disadvantaged in this block: s/he is not credited with the healing that s/he generates from within, and s/he is always regarded by the medical professionals as a potential victim of the mother's incompetence.

These relationships between professionals and layfolk will not be turned around by the professionals. This is not to say that there are not some medical experts who have overcome their training and the prevailing philosophy of professionalism — there are a few, and some are remarkably wise and helpful in their understanding of healthiness and healing. But for the most part medical professionals have no reason to change the way they deal with their patients.

Layfolk, on the other hand, have much to gain by altering their behavior with medical experts. If all of us understand that we are responsible for our own healing, we can learn to use professionals as resources for teaching. Mothers, as temporary agents for their children's health, can learn from medical professionals and in turn teach about healing to their children.

## A Concept of Health

It is important to remember that our expectations of medical experts, and their preference for dramatic rescue work, combine to present enormous obstacles to the invention of a concept of health. I invite you now to join in that invention, by focusing on the notion of a healthful life as the primary goal of our responsibility of mothering. The invention, the very concept of healthiness, should be seen as a *process*, a goal toward which we are working, a mode of understanding. As long as we see health as a *product* to be gained, or manufactured, or bought and sold, we are defeated by the evidence of our daily afflictions, for which we have no reason or understanding.

I believe that we can begin to see health as a *process* by:

- Reclaiming the *knowledge and skills* needed to cope with illness and injury and pain, at home and with the compassionate assistance of family, kin, friends, and neighbors. Most of the medical care provided right now, for a fee, by professionals, does not require lengthy education in special schools, or the use of complicated technology, or access to dangerous manufactured chemicals. It is based on some rather simple skills of examination, some rather simple principles of healing, and some rather simple skills and substances for treatment. Most of that kind of care can be learned by mothers and can be applied to children at home, with the supervisory assistance of medical experts.

- Learning to think about the *meaning of weakness, suffering, and affliction* in the course of human life. Is vomiting, for instance, always a symptom of nonhealth, to be stopped by chemical remedies as soon as it begins? Or is it a natural way of ridding the body of noxious or unneeded substances, a cleansing that allows our natural defenses to cope with an underlying affliction? Is fever a form of needless suffering, always to be beaten away with potentially hazardous chemicals, or might fever have some adaptive advantage in the body's struggle against infection or inflammation? What inner resources do we have to draw on when we are weak or injured or in pain? What growth and change can come to us through our struggles with affliction? If we hate and blame ourselves when we have symptoms of dis-ease, what do we feel about and teach to our children when *they* are ill? Are not adaptation to weakness and injury and pain, and coping with recovery and change and growth, evidence of the strengthening of one's underlying good health?

- Learning — or relearning, if we can remember our ancient human heritage — that *we are part of a natural order,* and that loving ourselves means also loving the plants and animals, the water and air and wind and stars, amongst which we are privileged to live. If we are not human *animals* — a part of that natural order — are we then human *machines* — a part of technology? Is a notion of health defined only as the absence of diseases a cruel hoax that makes us interchangeable counters in an industrialized universe of machinery and commerce? Where do we search first for the tools and substances we need for the restoration of our health when we are ill? Do we try to repair our machinery-bodies with electronic machinery and the manufactured products of technology, or do we apply to human hands and eyes and ken and to the simple substances that grow and exist in the natural world?

Children grasp our prevailing notions of illness at a remarkably early age. Most school-aged children, when asked about the causes of illness, bypass the explanations about infectious agents and deranged metabolism (which they have been told about in school) and get right to the heart of the matter: we become ill, they say, because we are negligent, or disobedient, or bad. They have learned our adult attitudes of guilt and self-blame. They do not say, for instance, "I get sick when my body needs a rest." Nor do they say, as is said in some other cultures, "I get sick when the bad spirits come into me." The range of treatments that we provide for our bodies when we feel bad is determined partly by our beliefs about the reasons for feeling bad. If one believes in spiritual causes, then part of the treatment will be spiritual supplication. If one believes that one should have stayed well except for personal negligence or failure, then part of the treatment will be self-punishment. If, on the other hand, one believes that the symptoms of dis-ease are our bodies' cries for attention, comfort, and rest, and that ministering to dis-ease promotes opportunities for coping and adaptational growth, then treatments will be applied in quite a different spirit. The actual treatment may be the same in each of these instances — for instance, an antibiotic to combat a specific bacterial infection — but the reasons, the mood, and the understanding that surround the treatment will be different in each case. And the outcome —

the kind of person who emerges healthy again — will be different.

Children also can learn, very quickly and easily, how to be caretakers for themselves and for others. Although children in our culture are early indoctrinated into the attitudes of good patienthood — they often say that what they should do when they feel ill is "ask Mommy" or "go to the doctor" — they can learn readily and with enthusiasm to make wise and self-determined decisions about their own bodies. They can learn how to make balanced decisions about their own complaints. Those active decisions can make a difference in their sense of well-being. Similarly, school-aged children can and do learn a variety of caretaking skills that allow them to cleanse and dress wounds, nurse a fever or vomiting, massage and comfort aches and sprains for themselves, for their friends, and for members of their own families. And almost all children, before the adult world teaches them differently, know with certainty that they have a kinship with other animals, growing plants, the food they consume, and the air they breathe. In some respects, then, our children are already holding doors open for us, and we need only insure that these doors not be closed so that we and they together can go through to explore a new sense of healthiness.

Being with children can, if we will allow, force us to reexamine some of our learned assumptions about our own lives. In our lives, we may have accepted what we have been taught about health as little more than a prolongation of life, a compatibility with the world of employed labor and machines, and a capacity to adapt to many inhuman changes. For our children, whom we have borne in joyous pain and nurtured with a palpable investment of caring and energy, we may hope for something more. If we are willing to accept the risks associated with professionalized medical treatment, we may yet want to weigh those risks more cautiously for our children. Healthful living for children and adults is not essentially different, as I understand it. We can learn as much from our children as we teach to them if we dare to explore, with them, the process of health.

# CHAPTER 2

# Taking a Health History

We wish to evolve a system of deciding how healthy a child is — the ways in which s/he is doing well and is strong and sturdy, and the ways in which s/he is likely to succumb to affliction and need to go through a healing process, with or without outside help.

Medical professionals usually see their clinical work as the assessment of illness. Diagnosis means literally "to know through" and carries a flavor of labeling categories of disease. Our intent — assessing healthiness rather than looking only for disease — has a different perspective. Concern for the healthiness of our children requires a complete picture of ease and dis-ease, strengths and weaknesses. Mothers, who know their children intimately and on a day-to-day basis, can know and understand — better than any distant professional — a child's basic sturdiness and special strengths.

## Dimensions of Healthiness

I find it useful to think about healthiness in four general categories:

*Serenity:* a peacefulness that enables one to become engaged in a variety of activities, in thoughts of the moment, in dreams and reveries, and in plans for the future. Serenity is also the absence of distraction or preoccupation with immediate distress or pain. It is the sense that "all is right" with one's body, and that one need not attend to it except to enjoy or appreciate.

*Function:* the smooth and harmonious procession of the natural occurrences of activity, rest, and repair of body, mind, self, and soul. Healthy function enables us to act, reflect, and interpret, supporting creative adaptation to the natural and social environment. Function means also the absence of distraction or preoccupation with insufficient, misdirected, or excessive activity or adaptation. It is the sense that one's body will carry out its own necessary and important processes, smoothly and efficiently, without special attention or assistance.

*Capability:* the ability to carry out one's usual activities, accommodations, and assimilations, and to stretch to new abilities not before achieved. Capability is the absence of distraction or preoccupation with ineptness or failure in one's attempts to carry out accustomed behavior.

*Beauty:* the external appearance of good health, brightness of eye, intactness of skin, the glow that reflects serenity, function, and capability. The beauty of a healthy, whole animal is very different from the "beauty" dictated by social or cultural convention. Beauty is also the absence of distraction or preoccupation with disfigurement. It is the sense that internal serenity and function and external behavior and appearance are in harmony.

For each of these manifestations of healthiness, it is important to remember that each individual child — just like each adult — possesses his/her own constitution, makeup, predisposition, talents, and configuration. Our science, the dominant philosophy of the medical profession, imposes on our thinking an addiction to the average, the normal, and the ideal. There is, in addition, a belief that we "really" know something if we can put a number to it. Numbering is often a pseudo-measurement, but once numbers are assigned it is difficult to resist the temptation to compare one number with another and to assign a value of good or right to some numbers out of the entire possible range of numbers.

Comparison against norms and averages is only one way — sometimes useful, but very limited — to assess healthiness. It results, again, in a negative definition of health — the absence of deviation from the average. In addition it ignores or denies the fantastic range of individuality in human form and function. The human body takes many forms and has finely detailed variations in its function. An awesome array of individual variation is compatible with serenity, function, capability, and beauty. We know this through our own sight, hearing, and touch. We have some very solid evidence about biochemical individuality that shatters the myth that we are all identical replicas on a single model, and the associated myth that variations from that model are in and of themselves marks of nonhealth. For instance, only some of us can enjoy and be nourished by milk after the period of infancy; we vary widely, after our early years, in our *natural* and individual levels of intestinal enzymes to digest milk. Despite this, most in-school feeding programs for poor children offer only a small variety of foodstuffs, of which milk is usually one, ignoring the fact that for many children milk is neither a pleasure to consume nor a useful source of nutrients.

One of our most important tasks as mothers is to come to know the individuality of each of our singular children — as best as one person can ever "know" another. For beyond some invisible space we are always outsiders, onlookers to each other, and can never know others — not even the children who came from our bodies — as we know ourselves. But as adults in intimate contact with our children we do have not only the opportunity but also the responsibility to try to know and understand them as best we can. Further, as they grow we have the responsibility of telling them how we see them, not only so that they can understand the perceptions that direct our behavior toward them but also so that they can correct our perceptions when those do not tally with their self-knowledge. The bundle of individualities and idiosyncracies that makes up each child needs to be observed, understood, and accepted as his or her authentic self. All assessments of healthiness proceed against those benchmarks.

## Dimensions of Dis-Ease

When we suspect that something is not right in the health of our children, when we sense that there may be a trivial or a major dis-ease, we must turn around our categories of health and look at the counterparts to serenity, function, capability, and beauty.

*Distress:* the experience of discomfort or pain or affliction. Pain, discomfort, and affliction can be perceived as arising from a variety of sources: from the realm of the physical, as when one's head throbs, or muscles ache, or the gut cramps; from the realm of thinking, as when new information conflicts with previous understandings or beliefs, or is uncomfortably surprising; from the realm of the emotions, as in anxiety, sadness, or anger; or from the realm of the spiritual, as when a child is pushed to anguish about the meaning of suffering.

*Dysfunction:* natural bodily processes that have gone wrong, are out of kilter, are excessive or deficient or unaccustomed. Common physical dysfunctions are vomiting, diarrhea, fever, breathing disorders like croupiness or wheezing, inefficient wound healing, inefficient clotting of the blood, and inability to ward off common everyday infectious agents, like cold viruses, to which we are usually somewhat resistant. For some persons, a *usual* state of function might result in disease. For instance, the hemophiliac — whose blood clots poorly and who is therefore subject to excessive bleeding as a result of injury — may restrict his/her activities in order to minimize injury, thus also bringing on a kind of disability.

*Disability:* weakness, an absence or reduction of agility or endurance, regression from a former level of capability, or a relative lack of adaptability to new situations or challenges. Disability in children is commonly seen as regression — losing, usually only temporarily, the ability to act in ways that have been recently learned. Disability can also appear as developmental lag — failing to progress in new ways that could be expected from a knowledge of the child's history. Developmental lag, as a kind of disability, can be distinguished from developmental plateau (a healthy and expected pause between spurts of maturity) only by observation over time. Again, the use of norms and averages ("this three-year-old child, who should be able to ride a tricycle because most three-year-olds can ride tricycles, is lagging in his/her development") risks the harmful consequences of pejorative labeling. The only justified use of norms and averages is as benchmarks to describe, with positive acceptance, the individuality of a singular child.

Disfigurement: an interruption of integrity or wholeness; a change in physical structure that results in a reduction of self-protection, vigor, or adaptability. Common disfigurements are lacerations and abrasions, bruises, weeping rashes, tumors that become unsightly, and loss of hair or severe weight loss or gain that displace one's image of one's self.

## Dimensions of Healing

It should be apparent that health is a process and that perfect healthiness is probably never attained. It is part of the human condition always to have some distraction to serenity, some lapse in function, some interference with capability, some imperfection in beauty. It is how we cope with these manifestations of dis-ease that comprises the health of the moment. Striving for health means striving to accept and respect ourselves so that it is possible always to keep moving toward serenity, function, capability, and beauty.

In assessing health, then, it is as important to consider strengths as it is to evaluate dis-ease. It is, I think, an important and very maladaptive aspect of the medical professional's ordinary habits of thinking about disease that the focus is only on problems and not at all on strengths. An alternate view is to regard the professional as a supporter of the strengths of the layperson. The professional simultaneously can act as a resource for temporary remedies and for information and instruction that can increase the layperson's capacity for self-healing.

In this light, we might consider the following, among others, as resources of strength and potential adjuncts to self-healing:

- The ability to *tolerate* distress, dysfunction, disability, and disfigurement without demonstrating anxiety, anger, or depression to a degree that is harmful to one's self and to others.
- The ability to *compartmentalize* dis-ease so that it does not envelope and weaken all of one's diverse strengths.
- *Adaptability* to change and new experience.
- The ability to *recognize* one's own needs.
- The ability to *ask for help* from others.
- A degree of *grace and acceptance* in affliction.
- Reserves of *energy and endurance.*
- A *sense of humor* that finds wry pleasure in the unaccustomed or the unexpected.
- The *patience* to await another day and new opportunities.
- *Flexibility* in the face of disrupted routines and lost expectations.
- Open *expression* of strong emotions (such as anger), without apprehension of punishment from one's self or others.
- A capacity to *struggle* with vigor against one's own self and against the world of people and circumstances outside one's self.
- *Acceptance* of one's self as worthy, effortful, and caring — even in the midst of affliction and dis-ease, even in weakness and disability, even through pain and disfigurement.

Children are not born with these strengths. They grope toward them tenuously, as plants grope toward the light. Mothers, also, find their own strengths failing or lost. We have the doubly difficult responsibility of maintaining our own strengths so that we can recognize and nurture the strengths of our children. It is also true that *their* developing strengths can make *our* tasks more difficult in some respects. Sturdy self-esteem, open expression of anger, stubborn endurance, and the patience to outwait are qualities that can simultaneously signal a strong child and a weary mother! And yet our responsibility is not only to get through this day but also to guide the child

to self-reliant, cooperative, caring adulthood. Mothers' sense
of humor about these matters is best shared with other mothers.

### "Taking a History" at Home

The mechanics of an assessment of health begin, as in the
diagnostic process used by doctors, by "taking a history." Most
doctors follow, in brief, outlines that they learned as part of
their medical training. The doctor works from the assumption
that the patient *will* have a disease, and that there will in all
likelihood be only one disease. The physician's diagnostic
process is thus very like that of the postal clerk who sorts mail
by hand, putting each item into one box or another and throw-
ing the few that cannot be categorized into a bin to be carted
off — perhaps someone else will attend to those, perhaps not,
but they are not part of the business at hand. Medical professionals will often admit to an analysis something like the following: this patient's complaints and findings do not really fit
into Category A or Category B, but they are more like Category
B than anything else, and I will so label and treat.

The health assessment that a mother can make for her
child offers some advantage over the diagnostic outline practiced by a doctor. Because a layperson is not limited by assumptions about disease categories, s/he is encouraged to describe the events surrounding the complaints and disorders in
question *as they were experienced by the child.* While there
may be lapses and holes in the interpretation of these events,
the events themselves are not filtered through or altered by the
pressure of fitting the situation into a predetermined category
of disease.

Whether a doctor is taking a diagnostic history or a mother
is assessing the state of her child's health, when the subject is
a child there are special efforts required in getting the needed
information. When the child is an infant and cannot yet speak
we must rely on observation and what we know about the
baby's usual behavior. For toddlers there is a much wider range
of behavior to consider; there are also the beginnings of language, usually very straightforward but limited in content and

expression. As children grow in the preschool years they develop a much more adequate language to describe their own internal events, but they also become canny about controlling themselves and others in their world. What they tell us then may be veiled or altered to gain special attention, to avoid taking a medicine, to ask for the ease of staying in bed or the privilege of running about with friends. In addition, there is still a good deal of uncertainty on the child's part about the proper words to use to describe the events of the body, as well as some spatial uncertainty about the location of those events. Older children are more expert in language and more skilled in describing bodily events. But they also tend to lose — unless we vigorously help them to retain — absolute certainty about and confidence in the sensations and signals that come from within.

Listening to messages from within can often be seen, for instance, in appetite and eating habits. Small children will take in a nutritiously balanced diet over a span of a week or two if they are offered an array of nutritious foods; they may eat only one thing on each day, but following their natural appetites — the signals of their bodies — they will choose a succession of foods so that their nutritional needs are met. We know that older children and adults modify their eating habits according to momentary relationships with people in their world, in response to foods that their friends eat and that they have seen advertised on TV or in grocery stores, or because of their own needs to be in control of what they put into their mouths. If we, as adults, forget our preconceived notions of what we should eat when we are ill and follow those dim signals of urge from our bodies, we usually can choose foods of an appropriate composition to aid in healing. But how dim, for most adults, those signals are! Sometimes parents can recapture their sense of their own bodily signals, and trust in their validity, as they strive to encourage their children to hold onto their confidence and respect for their own bodies' messages.

Following is a series of questions about health and disease. They are meant to be asked of the child if s/he is old enough to respond. For young children, the questions should be answered by anyone (including yourself) who has spent attentive time with them. Teaching children to consider and answer questions like these, as they mature in self-awareness, memory, and the ability to express such matters in words, is a key element of education for health.

This may appear to be a long list of questions. Once tried, it is clear that the answers to many of these questions are almost instantly self-evident. This is not to say that the process of assessing health and dis-ease is not time- and energy-consuming. In fact, one of the apparent advantages of going to a doctor for a diagnosis and treatment is just because that solution saves us a lot of work. But we also lose a great deal in that process.

*Serenity/Distress.* Do you hurt? Where? Is the hurt only in one small spot, or is it over a big area? Is it on the surface or underneath? Is it sharp like a knife or dull like a pressure? Does it go on all the time or does it come and go? When it hurts does it hurt the same all the time, or does the hurt get bigger and then smaller? When did it begin? What made it start? Can you do anything to make it go away? Can you do anything to make it hurt less? When it hurts, does it make you fall down, or stop playing, or be very still? Does it keep you from going to sleep? Does it wake you up? Have you ever had a hurt like this before? How did it go away then?

*Function/Dysfunction.* An understanding of the body's function is best gained by asking questions about the systems of the body affected.

- Eating and elimination. How is your appetite? Do you feel like eating right now? Do you think you will want to eat your supper? What would you like to eat? Are you thirsty? Have you vomited? How long after you ate did you vomit? What did it look like, the stuff that came up? Was there food in it? Anything that looked like blood? What had you been eating? Was there any green stuff in what you vomited? Does the vomit just come up, or does it really shoot out with great force? When did you last have a bowel movement? How often do you usually have a bowel movement? Was your stool hard or soft? What color was it — did you notice? Did it float in the toilet? Did it hurt when it came out? Was there anything in it that looked like blood? Have you had diarrhea? How often in the last day? When was the last time? Do you have diarrhea every time you eat? Does your belly hurt before you go? Does your mouth feel dry? Are you urinating as often as usual? When did you last urinate? (The last three questions are a check on whether the fluids lost in vomiting and diarrhea are very much in excess of the fluids taken in. Very young children may not know the word "urine." Such words as "pee" or "tinkle" may be more appropriate.)

• Breathing. Do you have a cough? Do you cough anything up? What does that look like? Does the cough feel deep in your chest or like a tickle in the back of your throat? Do you cough most when you first wake up in the morning? Do you cough most after you have been running and playing? Does the cough wake you up in the night? Has there been anything that looks like blood in the stuff you cough up? When did the cough begin? Is it different now than when it began? Are you having trouble breathing? Can you play as you usually do, or do you have to stop because you get short of breath? Do you have trouble breathing in? Do you have trouble breathing out? Have you ever had breathing trouble like this before? What happened just before the breathing trouble began? Does your ear hurt? Is there anything running out of your ear? Does it hurt when you wiggle your ear with your hand? Does your throat hurt? Does it hurt when you swallow? Do you want to eat anything? Do you want to drink anything? Are there lumps on the sides of your neck or under your chin? Do they hurt when you push at them? Are there any sores on your lips or in your mouth? Have you had a runny nose? Does it run from only one side of the nose, or from both sides? Is the stuff from your nose clear and watery, or yellow, or green? Does it have a bad smell?

• Urine system. Do you wet the bed? Do you ever have accidents in the daytime? Does it hurt when you urinate?

Do you go very often, a little bit at a time? Does it burn you when you urinate? Does your urine ever look red, or pink, or smoky? Do you drink more than other kids?

- The brain and other nerves. Do you have headaches? Where does your head hurt? What makes it start? Do you have headaches after you read or do close work? Do you know, before your headache starts, that you're going to have a headache? Do you vomit when you have a headache? Can you see all right? Can you see what the teacher writes on the blackboard when you sit at the back of the schoolroom? Can you see the leaves on the trees when you are walking down the street? Do you ever see two of something when there is only one? Can you hear things all right? Do you have any trouble hearing your teacher at school? Do you lose your balance or fall down a lot or bump into things when you don't expect to?

This is not an exhaustive list. There are other areas of questioning for the medical "review of systems." The systems reviewed above are, however, the most common areas of dysfunction for the kind of ailments that can be understood and remedied at home. Heart disease in children, for instance, is most commonly either a problem that the child is born with, or a problem that occurs after a severe illness. In either case, it is likely that a doctor will have listened to the child's heart with a stethoscope and heard a murmur — the most usual sign of heart disease in children. Those children with major heart disease are likely to have symptoms so marked — a blue color to the skin as a sign that the body is getting too little oxygen, or poor weight gain and slow development, or frequent and severe infections in the lungs — that they are almost certain to be taken to a doctor for diagnosis.

The preceding questions indicate the thoroughness of questioning (or, for the mothers of very young children, remembering and reflecting) that is needed to collect the necessary information to decide what is wrong with an ill child, and to decide whether the problem can be managed at home or a professional should be consulted from the start.

In addition to these questions, a mother can ask questions that deal with Capability/Disability. These questions might be answered by the child, by an older child for a younger one, or by an adult observer on behalf of the child. If answered by the child, the questions must be tailored to his or her age and developmental level.

*Capability/Disability.* Are you getting along with your friends about as well as you usually do? Are you getting along with your brothers and sisters about as well as you usually do? Do you play alone more often now than before? Do you get into more quarrels now than you used to? Are there things that you used to do that you don't want to do anymore? Do you get angry more often than you used to? Is school going as well as it used to? Do you get along with your teacher as well as before? Is your schoolwork harder for you than it used to be? Do you get tired more than you used to?

There are some questions that can be considered only by an observer and not by the child: Is the child playing in the same ways as before? In what ways is the child playing differently? Does the child seem more babyish than before? Is the child more quarrelsome, less tolerant, more solitary, more easily frustrated? Is the child more dependent, less self-determined, more attention-seeking, more defiant or sulky? Is the child more distractible, more careless, less interested, showing a shorter attention span, doing more daydreaming? Does the child get more easily fatigued, have less staying power? Has the child regressed from new habits (table etiquette, toilet training, and self-care like dressing and hair-combing) back to old ways? Is the child developing along at a steady rate, in terms of the new things s/he is learning to do, or has there been a leveling off or a slipping back?

*Beauty/Disfigurement.* Questions about the beginnings and characteristics of specific disfigurements — rashes, bruises, abrasions, dry skin, changes in hair or nails — can be asked of either child or mother. More general questions about overall appearance are difficult for anyone, child or adult, to answer about one's self and are best answered by the child's mother and other observers: Does the child look tired or heavy-

lidded much of the time? Does the child smile as often as
before? Does the child look fresh and rested after sleeping?
Does the child's skin color appear more pale or gray than
formerly? Have you noticed any remarkable changes, either
vague or specific, in the child's appearance?

For any new happening that might signal dis-ease, there
are four sets of general questions to ask. These questions can
help in deciding how to assist the process of self-healing.

- Appearance. What did this change look like in the beginning? How has it changed since then? Have you ever seen
  anything like this before?
- Time. When did it begin? Has it happened before? How
  long has it gone on? How has it changed over time? Has
  it been continuous or has it come and gone?
- Associations. Did it begin after any specific event? Did
  other changes occur at the same time? Might there be any
  relationship to foods that have been eaten or to materials
  or activities associated with school, with play, or with
  work? Were there stressful happenings just before or at
  the time this began? How has this change brought stress
  to the child? Might there be any relationship to travel to
  unfamiliar places? Has there been any exposure to known
  illness? Does anyone else in the family have complaints?
- Remedies. What makes the dis-ease better? What makes it
  worse? What has been tried to remedy the change? Has
  that helped? Has that made things worse? What does the
  child think would make the dis-ease go away?

## Family History

You should also review and note in writing your child's family
medical history. The following conditions run in families and
may have consequences for child health:

- Diabetes mellitus, especially that beginning in childhood.
  It is this form of diabetes that is most likely to be inherited.
  With a known instance of juvenile-onset diabetes (before
  age 20), your child should be observed more closely than

other children for evidence of inefficient metabolism of sugar. Urine tests for sugar should be done yearly and at times of acute illness. Occasionally a series of blood tests that demonstrate sugar metabolism over time (glucose tolerance tests) might be advised.

- Arthritis in childhood and rheumatic fever. The tendency to be afflicted with these illnesses runs in families.
- High blood pressure before the age of twenty. High blood pressure in children is rare, and is often associated with other disease conditions that are heritable. When several family members have high blood pressure your child's blood pressure should be measured yearly, and s/he should begin as a child a regimen designed to keep blood pressure down, including scant use of table salt and regular vigorous exercise.
- Heart attacks before the age of 45. When a family member has had a heart attack at such an early age there is sometimes an inherited condition of increased fats in the blood, a condition that can be discovered by laboratory test and controlled by diet.
- Other significant heart troubles. Congenital heart problems sometimes run in families, as does the tendency for rheumatic fever, mentioned above.
- Kidney disease. Some kinds of kidney disease are heritable.
- Easy bleeding. Various forms of bleeding tendency run in families; if one knows the specific type of bleeding disorder (discovered by laboratory tests of the blood) one can predict the probability that children in the family will have the same disorder.
- Sickle-cell anemia or other severe kinds of anemia. There are various inherited forms of anemia that can be discovered by laboratory tests.
- Allergies. The tendency to have allergic symptoms — hay fever, hives, eczema, and asthma — runs in families.
- Cystic fibrosis. This chronic disease, which causes respiratory and digestive problems, is inherited, can be diagnosed, and is treatable.

- Blindness and deafness. A few forms of these problems run in families.
- Babies who have died unexpectedly or of unknown cause. Sometimes this tragedy happens more than once in a family; often the cause is difficult to determine.
- Tuberculosis. This is not an inherited disease, but one that can lie dormant in an individual for many years and then erupt to give mild or severe symptoms. A child who is in contact with someone known to have had tuberculosis should be checked regularly by TB skin test.
- You should also take note of any other kinds of dis-ease that seem to occur on either side of your child's family.

**Categories of Illness**

For some dis-eases — actually relatively few — there are specific remedies. The healing of a throat infection with the bacteria called streptococcus, for instance, can be specifically helped by the antibiotic called penicillin. For most illnesses, however, the remedies that can be applied are supportive. They ease the discomfort of symptoms, or allow and assist the natural healing potential of the person who is ill for overcoming the dis-ease, or for coping with and adjusting to the existence of the malady.

The major practical purpose in deciding on a "diagnosis" — naming the kind of dis-ease that exists — is to decide on appropriate remedies to offer. The health review outlined in this chapter allows mothers to *describe* their children's disorders. Doctors are trained — indeed, obligated by the current conventions of medical practice — to *name* the disorder. As suggested earlier, doctors sometimes make diagnostic errors because they do not reach a full and detailed description of the picture they are striving to attain. For this reason, the kind of health review that has been outlined — a review to be conducted by a mother who already knows her child very well, and who can therefore focus on recent change or deviation from the child's usual and ordinary serenity, function, capability, and beauty — will produce a picture of the dis-ease that is full and comprehensible.

In order to make decisions about specific remedies, however, it is useful to group dis-cases into categories. Dis-ease and discomfort can be categorized in a variety of ways. The belief system of any culture includes a set of guidelines for differentiating one illness from another. We have our own belief system in our culture, and that belief system determines what we think are appropriate remedies. We do *not* believe, as do people from other cultures, that dis-eases can be caused by the visitation of spirits, by black magic practiced by enemies, or by the movement of celestial bodies.

We do, however, share a belief — largely unspoken — that we should have been able to keep ourselves or those we love from getting sick or hurt in the first place. (We should be aware that this responsibility — and this opportunity for feeling guilty — falls largely on women, for we are usually assigned and usually accept the responsibility of keeping those we love in good health.) Often our remedies, and the manner in which they are administered, are as much like punishments as they are like comforts.

Over and above our underlying belief that ill health should have been avoided and prevented and is therefore a cause for blame (especially self-blame) we have a belief system that categorizes dis-ease according to causes. We regard this as a "scientific" system. The "facts" on which that system is based are usually put forth with absolute assurance and then, often, said to be not true at some later date.

The important question for us is not whether our prevailing belief system about the categorization of dis-ease according to cause is ultimately valid or not valid. For us the important question is whether that system of classification helps us to decide on remedies that will help more than they harm.

For this reason it is useful, in considering home health care for children, to review the major accepted medical categories of dis-ease. Note that a full and accurate description of the events of the dis-ease will always be the central key to understanding the malady and selecting remedies. Sometimes, however, it is necessary to make an assumption about the category of illness in order to offer a remedy that might be most helpful.

The following list summarizes the major categories of illness according to our prevailing scientific belief system. The categories are grouped by similarity of cause:

*Disorders caused by nutritional aberrations.* Some maladies appear to result from eating too much or too little of some foodstuff. For instance, some now believe that the chronic ingestion of large amounts of refined sugar (probably the most prevalent addiction in our culture) can cause diabetes. The body becomes exhausted in its ability to respond to very high blood sugar. There are spells of low blood sugar, when the body overreacts to the presence of high blood sugar. Also, there are disabling swings of mood, attention, and alertness as the body alternates between periods of very high and very low blood sugar.

Specific conditions result from marked deprivation of specific vitamins and minerals. There are probably many other less well defined conditions that result from relative lacks of such nutrients, or from lacks of several such nutrients at once. Nutrient deficiencies can readily cause changes in the skin, hair, nails, and in the central nervous system — shown by changes in attention, coordination, steadiness, and the senses of touch, vision, and hearing. Excesses of certain foodstuffs may put a strain on the kidneys and bowels (excretion of waste), on the digestive organs (exhaustion or strain on the digestive juices and actions), and on the heart and blood vessels (changed composition of the blood). Excesses of some foodstuffs can result in deficiencies of other foodstuffs, by competition. Chronic deficiencies of major nutrients, such as protein, can result in a significant slowing of physical growth.

*Disorders caused by infection.* Some maladies appear to result from the invasion of the body by infectious organisms. These organisms can be viruses, bacteria, parasites, or other more obscure varieties like rickettsiae. Infectious organisms are passed along by other persons or by animals. Occasionally there is an intermediate host — that is, the organisms can pass from a person or animal to an eating utensil or an agent like an insect, from which someone else can be exposed and made ill. Usually, however, we catch infections directly from other people. The most common means of spread between people are by the respiratory tract (sneezing, coughing, kissing, breathing on, or sharing eating utensils or toothbrushes), by the digestive tract (especially through excretion — by stool contamination of the hands), or by direct skin-to-skin contact. Household and barnyard animals can sometimes be sources of infection, even when they themselves do not appear ill. Insects can also carry infection.

Infections can involve only one localized part of the body (as when bacteria infect the bladder, or middle ear, or the throat). Or infections can involve the bloodstream and can involve potentially every organ of the body — this is the usual case with viruses. Infections often but not always cause fever, and may also cause an enlargement of the lymph nodes, those structures in the body that make specific substances, antibodies, to combat the infectious agents.

*Disorders caused by tumors.* Tumors are either localized swellings that appear on the surface of the body or are masses that occupy space inside the body. Tumors inside the body usually push aside organs and cause symptoms by crowding or stretching. *Benign* tumors do not spread to other parts of the body. They cause symptoms only because they are disfiguring or because they take up space. They can be removed; sometimes their removal causes new dis-ease, as a consequence of surgery, X-ray, freezing, or cautery used for the removal.

Cancers are *malignant* growths. Not all malignant growths are swellings or tumors. Some, for instance, are growths in the bloodstream, like leukemia. Malignant tumors grow so that they spread away from the original site of growth and invade other parts of the body. Usually all parts of a malignant tumor must be removed in order to stop its growth. Tumors in children usually grow quite rapidly, compared to those in adults. . Some tumors are present, if only in seed form, at the time of birth. Others begin to grow at some later time in life. Most malignant tumors (cancers) are now believed to be caused by chemical pollution of our air, water, and foodstuffs usually produced by industrial and commercial contamination.

*Disorders caused by poisons.* Poisons in our environment cause not only cancers but also respiratory dis-ease and diseases of the blood, the nervous system, the skin, and almost every organ system. Poisons can change the metabolic system so that we cannot benefit from the nutrients in the foods we eat. Some poisons, like lead, can have instantaneous and severe effects. Poisons can also show their effects after long-term chronic low-level exposure, like the lead we breathe in from gasoline fumes. Most poisons are equally dangerous, whether taken in a single, very large dose or taken in small amounts over a long period of time. In addition to the poisoning effects of environmental pollution, poisoning accidents — usually at home — are frequent hazards for children. Many commercial household products, such as those sold for cleaning, are poisonous when ingested, spilled on the skin, or inhaled. Most medicines are poisonous when taken in overly large doses.

*Disorders caused by accidents.* Some accidents are almost unavoidable consequences of an active life, like a fall on the ice or an eye injury from a tree branch. Other accidents are peculiar to our industrialized way of life. The automobile, for instance, is by far the single most frequent agent in serious accidents to children. Accidents, poisoning, and nutritional disorders together make up the most common and serious causes of injury and illness in our children.

*Disorders caused by individual aberrations of metabolism.* There are some individuals whose inborn constitutions are such that their normal body functions are disabling or disfiguring. Examples are hemophilia (a tendency to bleed excessively) and PKU, or phenylketonuria (a condition of slow and limited motor and mental development). Other metabolic conditions can develop after birth and have similar consequences. Examples are diabetes mellitus (a limited ability to process sugar in the bloodstream) and hypothyroidism (a limited supply of the hormonal substance used in most of the body's energy transactions.) In this area modern medicine has devised some effective treatments for truly disabling or even life-threatening conditions. On the other hand, the existence of effective treatments sometimes induces medical experts to call us sick when our constitutional individuality is only mildly disabling and we are quite capable of living normal lives.

*Disorders caused by allergy.* There are major individual variations in our bodies' tendencies to react to allergenic substances. Some of us react promptly, frequently, and severely to contact with substances that our bodies identify as foreign and presumably dangerous. Others seem to have virtually no allergic tendencies, although it is likely that an appropriate allergenic stimulus could produce at least a mild allergic reaction in anyone. Witness the many children who have boastfully tried to demonstrate that *they* couldn't get poison ivy by rubbing themselves all over with the leaves — only to induce a massive and uncomfortable allergic reaction. In the allergic reaction the body produces a rush of chemicals to fight off the substance that is recognized as foreign. This foreign substance may be something eaten, something breathed in, something in contact with the skin, or something injected by an insect or a needle. The chemicals that the body produces actually cause the symptoms. The symptoms of an allergic reaction may range from something so mild as a chronic drippy nose to a life-threatening combination of spasms of the larynx (interfering with the ability to breathe) and shock (a marked fall in the blood pressure that interferes with the essential supply of oxygen to the brain). The degree of distress, dysfunction, disablement, and disfigurement needs to be considered carefully, for this is another area in which one can easily be induced to become a sick patient. One would not want to make innumerable visits to clinics and doctors and accept frequent treatments for symptoms that are in fact mild and cause little real disease.

*Disorders caused by stress.* The body reacts to stress (events that we perceive and then interpret to be stressful) with a complex set of changes intended to prepare us for fight or flight. A concentration of stressful events — that is, events that a given individual perceives and interprets as stressful — can cause a wide range of symptoms, including some kinds of distress, dysfunction, disability, and disfigurement. While the bodily reaction can be prevented or corrected by some very powerful and potentially dangerous chemical, medicinal substances, it is more sane to try to alter the source of the stressful events, or to alter the individual's reaction to those events so they are no longer perceived as stressful but as something that can be coped with.

The information gained from a questioning of the child, one's self as the child's parent, and others will produce a description of the disorder and the events surrounding its appearance. For some of the common childhood disorders, a mother can readily learn to recognize and interpret these events and to decide what is right and what is wrong with her child's health.

It is well to keep the written record of all home-based information about your child's health in a file or notebook. At some later date your observations may be of critical importance to you or to a medical professional in understanding your child. Since it is difficult to know just what bit of information may be useful at a later time, it is probably better to take complete rather than scanty notes.

In this chapter we have been thinking mostly about the child's subjective experience of health or dis-ease. These *symptoms* are reported by the child telling what it is like to feel this way or that, how s/he got to this state, and what experiences seem to be related to the present state. While your child is very young his/her subjective experience must be interpreted by you, since s/he is not yet adept at reporting such matters. In the next chapter we will consider *signs* of health and dis-ease, signals about the child's present state that can be observed objectively by you or anyone else — including the child — who cares to look, feel, listen, taste, and smell.

# CHAPTER 3

# The Physical Examination

Every body looks and works a little differently from all others. No one of us is just the same as another.

It seems a little foolish to have to state this so baldly. But it is especially true with our children that we worry about small differences and little bits of individuality. With the recent prominence of cosmetic surgery we can feel compelled to straighten feet, shorten noses, pull back ears, and lift eyelids to make each person look like every other.

This attitude applies to bodily functions, also. Some of us burn sugar in such a way that, if we eat only three meals, we have spells of very low blood sugar. This kind of hypoglycemia is easily remedied by learning what and how to eat to make ourselves feel good through the day. We are sometimes inclined to think of this as an illness and to wonder if there are medicines that should be taken. Similarly, some children have relatively short attention spans well into the school years and are called hyperactive. It can be tempting to think of such children as "sick" and want to give them a medicine, when in many instances handling them differently until they mature will resolve any problems.

Several years ago I was directing a clinical service to diagnose (really, to describe) the functioning of children in their families. Our purpose was to find community-based help for their troubles. I worked at that time with a superb and talented clinical psychologist who tested the children.

She and I were fascinated by minor variations in the per-
formance of intellectual tasks by children whose total scores
were roughly equivalent. She began to explain these differences to the children, in a manner that conveyed her approval.
"I can tell by these tests that you like to work with numbers.
You are also very good at solving problems. But you have sort
of a hard time describing things in words. Lots of kids are like
that — and some are just the other way around. It's OK to be
either way — people are just different in those ways. You
should feel really good about doing well with numbers and
problems. And we'll see if your teacher and your mom and I
can figure out how to help you learn to describe things better
with words."

She and I were both pleased at the enormous sense of
relief that many children showed. It was as if they knew those
things about themselves and were glad that someone else knew
them too. They acted as if knowledge of their varied kinds of
capabilities had been held in, like a guilty secret. Perhaps their
teachers or parents had given a message that they were supposed to be "medium good" at everything. They seem to have
worried that there was something wrong with being especially
capable in one way and not so capable in another.

In the same way, I see parents in my pediatric practice
who worry about their child's uniqueness. They wonder if
there are medical (that is, sickness) labels to attach to accept-
ably healthy children who only deviate slightly from what has
been described as usual or average.

Any one body is best known and understood by the person
who lives in it. Children — until they are told not to — will
vigorously and enthusiastically poke, prod, feel, taste, smell,
and look at every part of their own bodies. As we adults know
only too well, someone often tells a child that that is vain, that
some parts are dirty, or that it is simply not nice to explore
oneself in that way.

We could, instead, help them to understand and recognize
what they are learning about themselves in that sort of explo-
ration. After the child, probably the one person who is most
likely to "know" a child's body is his/her mother. As we take

care of our children we hold them, caress them, kiss and hug them. All of our touching, looking, sniffing, and tasting gives us opportunities to know the configuration and details of their bodies. Often most of what we know is there in our heads but not thought about in any very organized or useful fashion.

Some of us shy away from this manner of knowing our children, as we were earlier taught not to know our own bodies. I recently saw a nine-year-old boy with an abdominal tumor that was far advanced. When I first saw him he was lying on a hospital bed; as I stood at the door of his room I could see from that distance the swelling and the outline of his tumor. He lived in a family of great physical modesty and personal distance. Family members rarely touched one another. He came to the clinic for a checkup before school began. The family had been together, just before that, at a lake on vacation. They had been wearing swimming suits and playing together, but because they rarely looked at each other's bodies and seldom touched each other's bare skin they were unaware of his tumor. Had others in the family looked at or touched him they could have known about his tumor, sought medical consultation, and perhaps saved his life.

Once again, as we learn the importance of knowing how well we understand our children's bodies, we adults have an opportunity to relearn what we knew when we were small children: that our own bodies are fascinating, infinitely wonderful, and different from all others. As we help our children recognize and interpret the information they have about themselves, we also transfer to them what we know about them. We can and should know enough about our children to enable them to find out and understand more about themselves. This role as knower of the child's body is only temporary. We increasingly transfer what we know to the child. In the end we are left with a residue of memories, finally of warm delight but of no practical application, of that very intimate job of being a mother.

Most of us would readily admit that we can never know another as well as we can know ourselves. We sometimes find ourselves believing that good parents should know *everything*

about their child — and of course we cannot, even must not.
There are subtle limits to our invasions of the child's person
and privacy — even the infant's — that we cannot violate. But
what we do know we must not deny, and what we can learn
in the course of mothering we should not shy away from.

In the ordinary course of mothering we can explore a
child's body in three related but different ways:

- Much of what we know we do not think about in any
  conscious fashion; it has been accumulated over years of
  touching and looking, tasting and smelling. That information is available for us to think about in an organized
  and collected fashion, if we choose to do so.
- At intervals — at least once a year, more frequently for
  young infants, and when we are uncertain of our skills
  — we should go through a planned physical examination,
  intently thinking about all that we already know and ex-
  ploring the child's body with all of our senses, in a
  thoughtful and formal manner.
- At any time when we want to review a health assessment
  we should reexamine those parts of the child's body that
  may have changed. This we might especially want to do
  when we wonder if, or in what manner, a child is ill.

## A Formal Physical Examination

The section that follows is an outline of a formal physical
examination of a child. Rarely does one need to put a child to
a lengthy inspection at one sitting, although some children
might enjoy such attention. Most of what needs to be known
will already be known. One only needs to think about that
knowledge, to look more closely, to feel some parts more intently, to conduct a formal review.

A few instruments are suggested for use in the physical
examination: a stethoscope, blood-pressure cuff, and otoscope.
Other materials are suggested for doing simple laboratory tests
of the throat, blood, and urine. These instruments and supplies
are easily purchased but are not inexpensive. They can be
bought and shared by a group of neighbors; by a day-care

center group; or by a neighborhood house, community center, or church organization.

Being able to use the instruments effectively may take some time. Certain techniques will need to be mastered. All the techniques are easy to learn, but don't hesitate to discuss the instruments or techniques with a doctor, nurse practitioner, or other health professional.

*Vital signs.* A formal health review always begins with measurements of the vital signs — height, weight, head circumference for babies under 18 months, pulse, respiration, blood pressure, and temperature.

- Height and weight. You should ask the doctor or nurse at your clinic for your own copy of the growth chart appropriate for your child's age and sex. There are four: one for infant boys, one for infant girls, one for older girls, and one for older boys. Growth charts are less useful for adolescents, since the charts show *averages* for each age and every child goes through her/his adolescent growth spurt at an individualized age and over an individualized period of time.

To measure and record weight, you should check your scales first to be sure that no weight registers as zero pounds. Always weigh the child nude if you want accurate weights for comparison. Remember that all scales have some expected error; with ordinary home scales the child's true weight is probably within two pounds more or less of the weight you read on the scale.

Record the weight on the chart by finding the point where the child's age (read across the bottom of the chart) intersects with the child's weight (read up and down the left-hand side of the chart).

Until a child can stand straight and still, one must measure height with the child lying on a flat surface. This is a very imprecise way to measure because you can measure the child twice in one day and the two measurements can differ by as much as an inch.

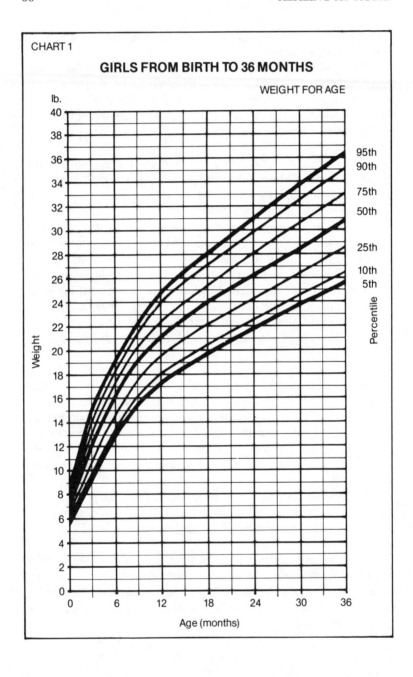

CHART 1

**GIRLS FROM BIRTH TO 36 MONTHS**

WEIGHT FOR AGE

lb.

95th
90th
75th
50th
25th
10th
5th

Percentile

Weight

Age (months)

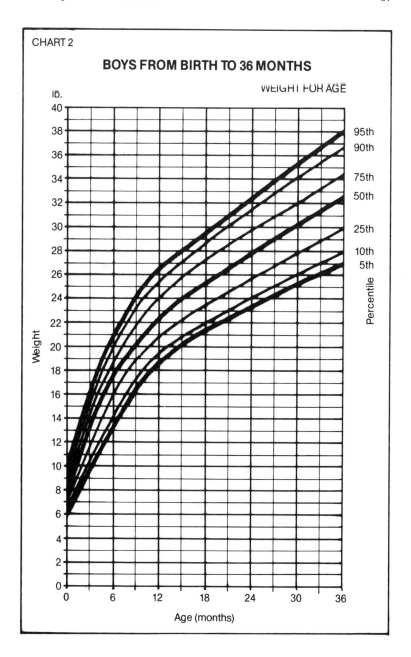

CHART 2

**BOYS FROM BIRTH TO 36 MONTHS**

WEIGHT FOR AGE

lb.

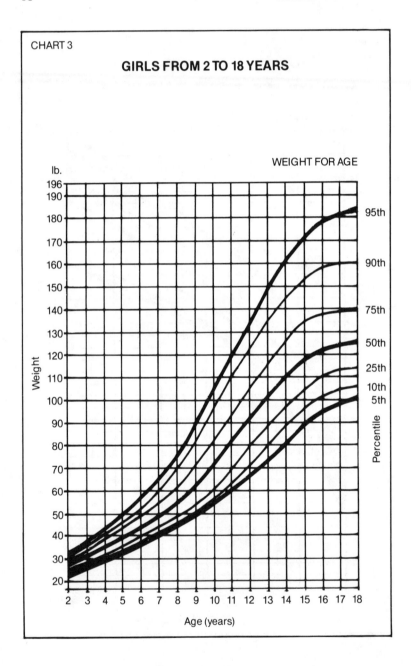

CHART 3

**GIRLS FROM 2 TO 18 YEARS**

WEIGHT FOR AGE

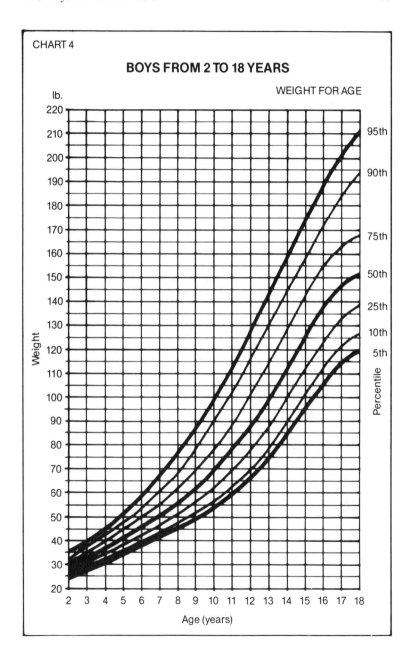

CHART 4

**BOYS FROM 2 TO 18 YEARS**

lb.                                              WEIGHT FOR AGE

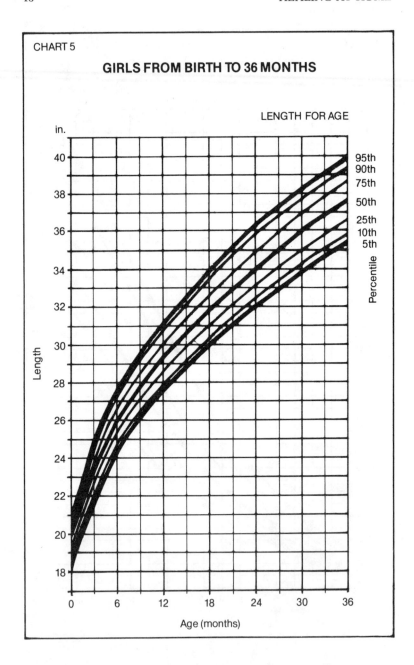

CHART 5

**GIRLS FROM BIRTH TO 36 MONTHS**

LENGTH FOR AGE

in.

40
38
36
34
32
30
28
26
24
22
20
18

Length

0    6    12    18    24    30    36

Age (months)

95th
90th
75th
50th
25th
10th
5th

Percentile

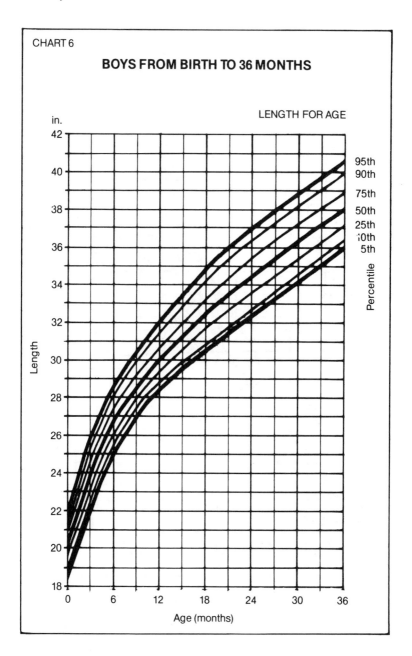

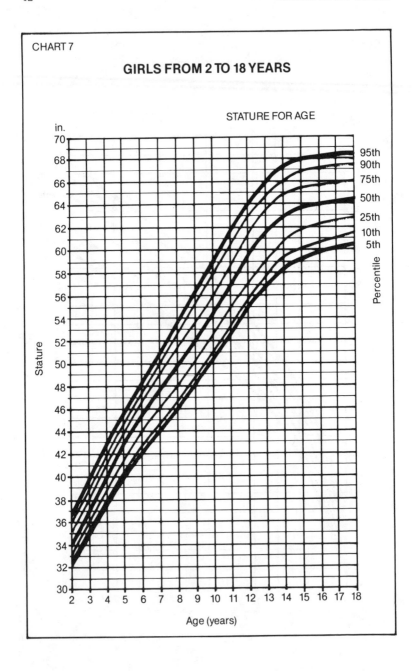

CHART 7

**GIRLS FROM 2 TO 18 YEARS**

STATURE FOR AGE

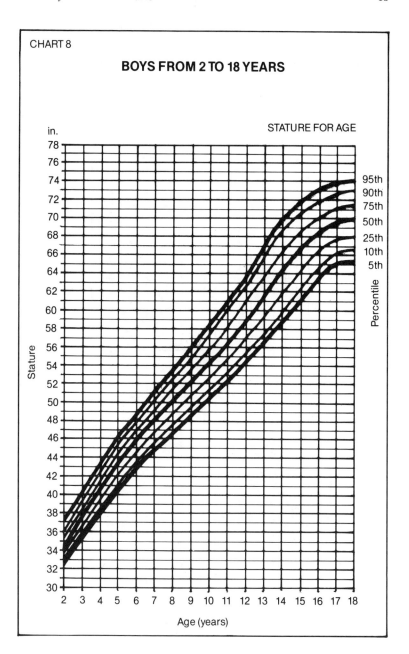

CHART 8

# BOYS FROM 2 TO 18 YEARS

in.

STATURE FOR AGE

Percentile

95th
90th
75th
50th
25th
10th
5th

Stature

Age (years)

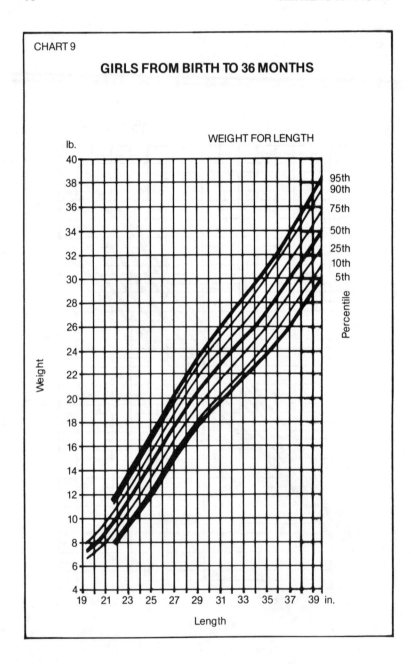

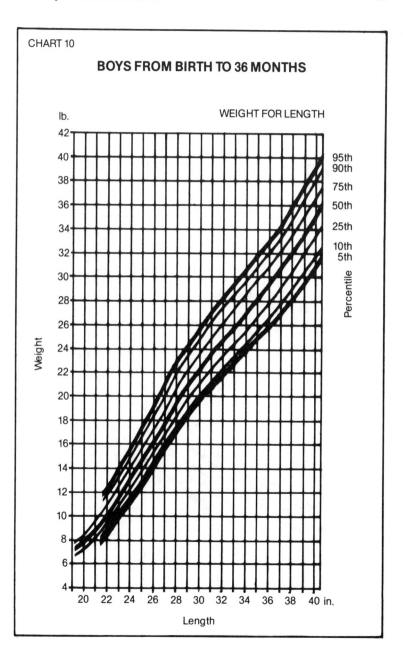

CHART 10

# BOYS FROM BIRTH TO 36 MONTHS

WEIGHT FOR LENGTH

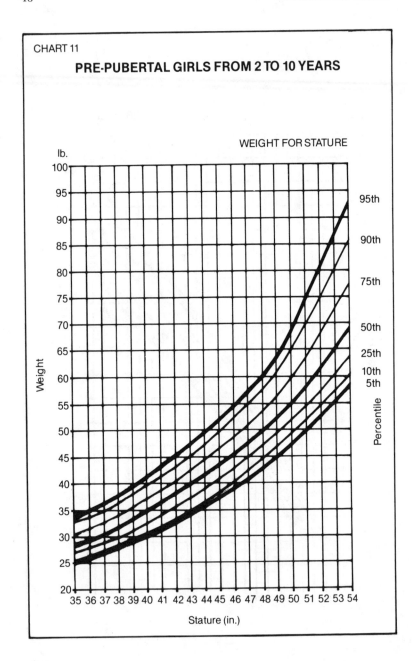

CHART 11

**PRE-PUBERTAL GIRLS FROM 2 TO 10 YEARS**

WEIGHT FOR STATURE

lb.

Weight

Stature (in.)

Percentile

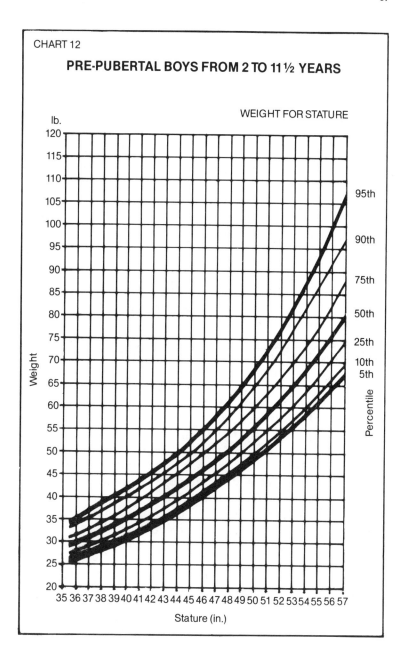

CHART 12

**PRE-PUBERTAL BOYS FROM 2 TO 11½ YEARS**

WEIGHT FOR STATURE

The child should be lying on her/his back on a flat surface, looking upward, with the top of the head against a wall or something similar. While one person holds the child's head in position, a second person holds the knees together, pushes them gently to the floor, and measures from the top of the head to the bottoms of the feet.

This measurement is recorded on the chart in the same fashion as weight was recorded. Always use the birth-to-36-month chart for height if the child was measured lying down.

When the child can stand straight and still, measure height against a wall. Glue a tape measure to the wall, or mark the point of the child's height with a pencil and later measure the distance from floor to point with a yardstick. The child's face should be forward, the heels up against the wall and the knees straight, not bent. This method of measuring height is somewhat more reliable than the method with the child lying down, although there is still some expected error in the measurement.

If the child's height has been measured with the child standing, record the height on the 2–18-year chart.

To record weight for length, make a mark on the chart at the point where length (read along the bottom of the chart) intersects with weight (read up and down along the sides of the chart.)

The important aspect of plotting heights and weights on a growth chart is that each child is expected to stay in a groove. Big children, who are at the upper end of normal, should follow an upper track of the curve, and small children are expected to stay in a lower track. Any marked change — a plateau of growth in weight or in height, or a fall in weight, or a sudden spurt in height or in weight — is worthy of notice, even though it may not mean that anything is wrong. To notice change over time we must keep a record over time.

After infancy, children ordinarily grow only in spurts. Mothers are sometimes confused by the marked variations in a child's appetite beginning at about 15 months. When children are not in a growth phase they eat little, for they are small people and need very few calories for weight maintenance. Just before a growth spurt they are likely to increase their appetites. Children rarely lose weight except when they *severely* limit intake or when they are seriously ill. (On the other hand, a child who is somewhat obese can slim out by holding weight steady, by reducing the calories in tho diot and waiting for the natural gain in height.)

It is now generally thought that obese babies, with weight in a significantly higher track than height on the growth chart, will likely be obese adults. It appears that they have not only more fat cells but larger fat cells than slim babies. While we mothers cannot entirely control our children's fatness or slimness, we can certainly influence their dietary intake toward relatively low-fat and low-sugar foodstuffs.

- Head circumference. Head-circumference norms are included on the standard growth charts. As with height and weight, it is the *rate* of growth that is important. This means that several measurements over time must be taken. One measures around the widest part of the head, from the bump at the back of the head (the occiput) around to the forehead.

- Pulse. There are only two common circumstances of significant pulse variation in children. The pulse rate increases in times of stress (as with a fever, or after exercise or excitement) and when there is significant anemia. Pulse rates are usually measured at rest. In general, the better one's physical condition the slower the pulse rate. A slow pulse rate can indicate heart or brain disease, but only when it is different from a child's usual rate, or when it is slower than the range of rates shown in Chart 15. The pulse should be regular, although children's pulses often quicken with inspiration (breathing in) and slow with expiration (breathing out). Pulse is usually measured for one minute, although it can also be measured for a longer time and averaged for one minute. The pulse can be felt with fingertips at the temple, the wrist, and on the top of the foot. It can also be measured by placing your ear (or a stethoscope) over the child's heart. Chart 15 shows average pulse rates for children of different ages.

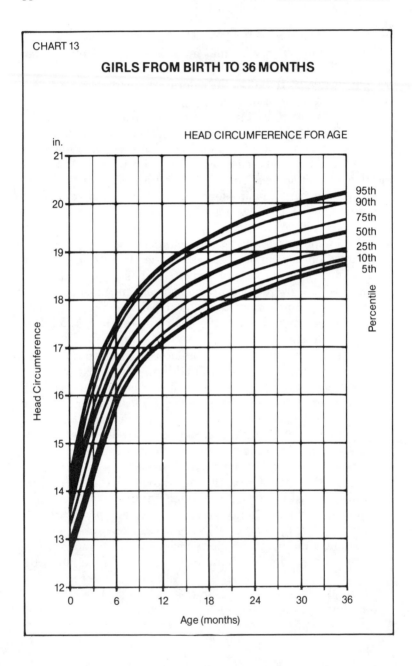

CHART 13

**GIRLS FROM BIRTH TO 36 MONTHS**

HEAD CIRCUMFERENCE FOR AGE

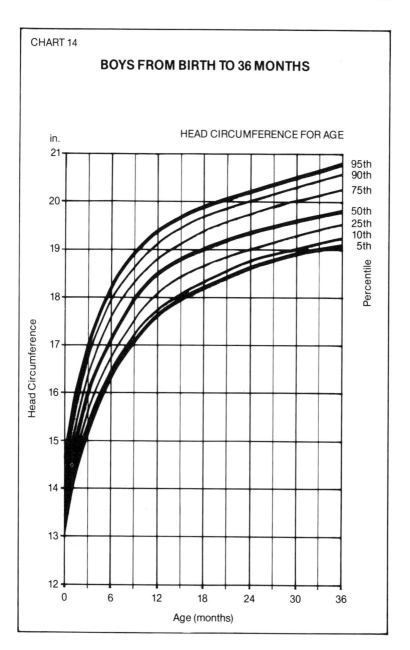

CHART 14

**BOYS FROM BIRTH TO 36 MONTHS**

HEAD CIRCUMFERENCE FOR AGE

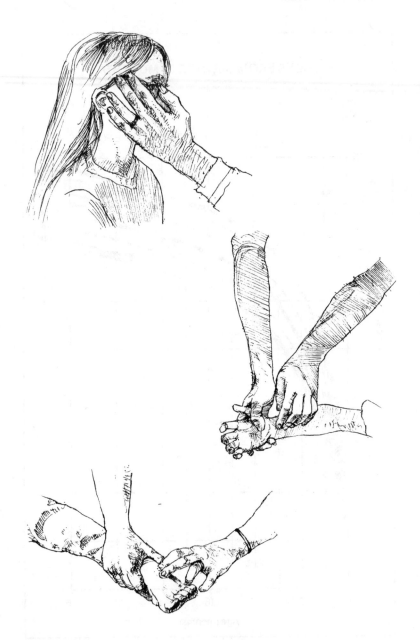

Feeling the pulse at the temple, wrist and foot

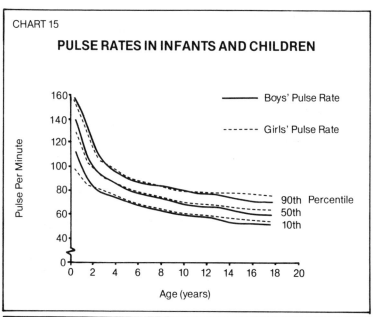

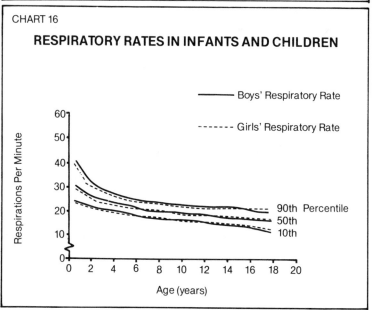

Both from: Nelson, Vaugham, McKay *Textbook of Pediatrics*, 9th Ed., 1969, W.B. Saunders, Phila.

- Respiration. The most common change in respiration occurs when it speeds up at times of stress, exercise, respiratory-tract infection, or fever. Respiration should be measured at rest and for a period of one minute. Chart 16 shows average respiratory rates for children of different ages.
- Blood pressure. It is difficult, and probably not practical at home, to measure blood pressure in a child who is too young to cooperate in the measurement. Some children will cooperate at the age of two, and others not until they are five or so.

High blood pressure often runs in families, and in these families even young children may have persistent blood-pressure readings that are a little high for their age. In families where it is known that parents or grandparents have high blood pressure, it is important to take the child's blood pressure on a yearly basis.

CHART 17

## NORMAL BLOOD PRESSURE FOR VARIOUS AGES

| AGES | MEAN SYSTOLIC ± 2 S.D. | MEAN DIASTOLIC ± 2 S.D. |
|---|---|---|
| Newborn | 80 ± 16 | 46 ± 16 |
| 6 mos.–1 year | 89 ± 29 | 60 ± 10 |
| 1 year | 96 ± 30 | 66 ± 25 |
| 2 years | 99 ± 25 | 64 ± 25 |
| 3 years | 100 ± 25 | 67 ± 23 |
| 4 years | 99 ± 20 | 65 ± 20 |
| 5–6 years | 94 ± 14 | 55 ± 9 |
| 6–7 years | 100 ± 15 | 56 ± 8 |
| 7–8 years | 102 ± 15 | 56 ± 8 |
| 8–9 years | 105 ± 16 | 57 ± 9 |
| 9–10 years | 107 ± 16 | 57 ± 9 |
| 10–11 years | 111 ± 17 | 58 ± 10 |
| 11–12 years | 113 ± 18 | 59 ± 10 |
| 12–13 years | 115 ± 19 | 59 ± 10 |
| 13–14 years | 118 ± 19 | 60 ± 10 |

From: Nadas & Fyler, *Pediatric Cardiology*, 3rd Ed., 1972, W.B. Saunders, Phila.

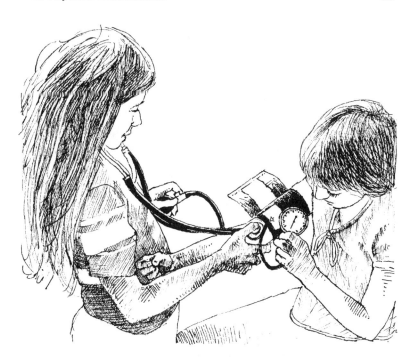

Measuring blood pressure

Blood pressure also rises in some relatively common children's diseases, especially diseases of the kidney. That is another good reason for knowing what your child's blood pressure usually is.

To measure blood pressure, one needs a stethoscope and a blood-pressure cuff. A nurse stethoscope can be bought for $10–15 from a medical-surgical supply house. Blood-pressure cuffs cost about $50.00 and have different-sized cuffs to measure blood pressure in people with different-sized arms. The cuff should be as wide as two-thirds of the length of the upper arm. The cost of a blood-pressure cuff and measuring dial (a sphygmomanometer) is such that several families could easily buy and share the use of a single set.

A blood-pressure cuff is a long cloth band that wraps

around the upper arm. Inside the cuff is a rubber bladder. It fills with air when you pump the bulb that is attached to the bladder. When the cloth band is wrapped securely around the arm and the bladder is filled with air, the flow of blood in the artery is stopped. As the air is slowly let out of the bladder, the blood starts to flow again. Blood flows in a pulse in the arteries, rather than in a steady stream, as in the veins. As you let the air out of the rubber bladder (by unscrewing, just a little, the screw that controls the rubber bulb), it is possible to hear, with a stethoscope, the sounds of the spurts of blood through the artery to the lower arm. To do this, you place the flat part of the stethoscope over the artery at the inside of the elbow; you find the place by feeling with your fingers for the pulse in the elbow before you fill the bladder with air. With the earpieces of the stethoscope in your ears, you listen carefully as you let the air slowly out of the rubber bladder. When you first hear a pulse (thump, thump, thump) you notice the reading on the dial; for an adult it would be about 120, but for a child it will be lower, depending on the child's age. When you don't hear the pulse anymore, you notice the reading again. The first reading is the systolic pressure; the lower reading is the diastolic pressure. Blood pressure is expressed as systolic over diastolic; for an adult an average reading is something like 120 over 70.

The standard deviation (S.D. on chart) is a way to indicate the expected range of variation in a blood-pressure reading. It should be interpreted in this way: For a four-year-old, the higher (systolic) measure of blood pressure should fall between the range of $99 - 20$ (79) and $99 + 20$ (119). If the systolic pressure of a four-year-old is less than 79 or higher than 119 this is very unusual and may indicate serious disease. Most four-year-olds will have a systolic pressure close to 99.

Many of us increase our blood pressure when we are nervous or anxious. It is always a good idea to take the blood pressure again if it seems high and you wonder if the child is a little nervous about having it taken.

- Temperature. This is the vital sign that mothers measure most often. There are several times when it is good to know what a child's temperature is. At the beginning of an illness, when you are wondering if the child might be ill, it is a good idea to measure the temperature accurately with a thermometer, since none of us is very exact with the time-honored mothers' technique of laying the back of a hand or a cheek against the child's cheek or forehead. When you know that the child has a fever and is ill, there is little point in taking the temperature again except perhaps to document how high the temperature is; since some kinds of illness are more likely to give a high fever, and others to give a low fever, it is often helpful to know exactly how high the fever is to decide what kind of illness the child has. You need not take the temperature again, in most illnesses, until you think that the child is getting better, when you may want to document that the fever is going down. In the end you will want to take the child's temperature again to be sure that the fever has gone away and thus it is reasonable to let the child up, out of the house, back to school, and in the company of his/her friends.

Body temperature can be measured by mouth, by rectum, or in the armpit. An armpit temperature (taken by holding the bulb of the thermometer in the child's armpit, with the upper arm held firmly against the side of the child's chest) is useful only for newborns, when we don't want to risk hurting the infant's rectum with the bulb of the thermometer. A normal armpit temperature is 36.4°C/97.6°F.

Rectal temperatures are taken past the newborn period until the time when a child can hold the bulb of the thermometer under the tongue, which is usually at about age five. Rectal temperatures are taken with a thermometer that has a round (not pointed) bulb. A rectal thermometer can be used to take the temperature by mouth (after it has been well washed and disinfected, of course) but an oral (by-mouth) thermometer cannot be used in the rectum, so if you have only one thermometer and a small child it makes more sense to have a rectal thermometer. To take a temperature by the rectum, lay the child across your knees, stomach down. Grease the end of the thermometer well with petroleum jelly, wipe a little petroleum jelly on the child's anus, and insert the thermometer about three quarters of an inch. Hold your hand across the child's buttocks, with the thermometer loosely between your fingers, and restrain the child (if s/he is wriggling) with your other hand. Keep the thermometer in for one minute, then take it out and read it. Insert it again and keep it in for one more minute, then read again. If the level has not changed, you have an accurate reading; if it has gone up (it will not go down, unless you shake it down), then you should continue to reinsert the thermometer for one-minute intervals until it stays at the same reading for two consecutive insertions. Normal rectal temperature is 37.6° C/99.6° F.

With most children over the age of five, the temperature can be taken by mouth. Again, it is sufficient to check the level of the mercury after the thermometer has been in the mouth for one-minute intervals; the lips must be kept closed around the thermometer. The normal temperature-reading by mouth is 37° C/98.6° F.

The following outline lays out a practical approach to a formalized physical examination of a child. Note that much of what you would learn by doing a complete physical examination of a strange child you will already know about your own child. There are several resources in the library, or that you might purchase for your own use, that will help you to interpret what you see and feel. Most importantly, ask nurses, doctors, and other medical experts to help you learn to examine your child.

*The head.* A newborn's head often has ridgy lumps. These are places where the edges of bones are riding up over other bones, as a result of the squeezing of the baby's head that always happens as the baby goes through the birth canal. There are two other kinds of lumps on newborn's heads that are, if not usual, at least not likely to give any real trouble. One is a cephalhematoma (literally, "a mass of blood on the head"). This results from bleeding under the thin membrane that covers the flat bones of the head. It can form as a consequence of the passage through the birth canal or because of manipulations that might have been done to help the baby out. This mass of blood will have edges that correspond to the outline of the bone that it lies over. It should disappear within a few weeks after birth. Sometimes a deposit of calcium is laid over its surface and it gets a thin, crunchy feel. In this case it will be somewhat slower to disappear altogether. The other kind of newborn head lump is a caput succedanum (literally, "the following head"). It is also a kind of bruise, but this time it is just under the scalp. It should go away entirely in a few days to weeks.

At birth there are two open spaces where the growing bones come together. One is at the crown, toward the front. The other (which is smaller, only fingertip size) is high on the back of the head. These two spaces, called fontanels, will close later as the bones grow to accommodate the infant's rapidly growing brain. The membrane that lies just under these open spaces is about as tough as cotton canvas.

After the age of about two, the bones grow together at their edges and the brain has reached about 90 percent of its adult size. Further brain growth will be accommodated by bone growth from the middle areas of the bones. By age two the head will have reached a shape that will not change greatly into adulthood. Before this time the bones of the head have been soft (mostly cartilage) and the head shape can easily be deformed, as it often is in the process of birth and as it can be when a baby lies mostly in one position (when one side might become flattened). After the age of two most of the lumps, bumps, and irregularities of the head will remain as that person's distinctive head shape.

In the back of the head, called the occiput, is the area of the brain where visual information is organized. Along the sides, toward the top, are the areas that send messages to all the nerves that make the muscles work, and the areas that receive the messages from all the nerves of skin and organ sensation. At the forehead or frontal area is the part of the brain that carries on the most complex thinking.

*Hair.* There are striking individual differences in the color and texture of hair. Most of the first growth of hair, that which is on the baby's head at birth, wears off rather quickly. The second growth then remains, to be changed slowly, over years, as the child grows.

Each hair has tiny barbs or projections. Hair that snarls easily probably catches itself on those barbs. The tendency to snarl and mat is usually a lifelong characteristic except that as one matures one's hair also becomes coarser, which can ease the tendency to snarl.

The skin of the scalp, like all skin, needs some exposure to fresh air to remain healthy. Small babies, especially those with blond hair, often have a condition called seborrhea, or partial blockage of the glands of the skin that produce sebum, a greasy, tallowlike substance that lubricates the skin. Seborrhea in older persons is called dandruff; seborrhea in babies is usually called cradle-cap. Untended, it will result in a layer of yellow, greasy scales overlying the scalp, preventing the scalp from contact with the air. While cradle-cap is not a disease, it can easily be cleared away to leave a healthier scalp.

The character of the hair, like that of skin and nails, reflects nutrition in a straightforward way. Skin, hair, nails, and the nervous system all are derived from the same embryonic source, called the ectoderm; all are very sensitive to nutritional adequacy. Hair and nails can be banded with growth corresponding to periods of altered nutrition. Hair and nails also take in some kinds of poisons, especially the heavy metals like lead.

Finally, hair is sensitive to stress. It can slow in its growth, fall out more than usual, or break off in patches (sometimes close to the scalp) in response to a child's experience of stress.

*Eyes.* The eyes reflect healthy beauty in a very special way. An ill child may have a heavy-lidded appearance. There is also a brightness or dullness of the eyes that has defied scientific description. It may reflect in part the serenity of the person looking out through those eyes.

The eyes display one of the "vital signs" of primitive and

essential central nervous function: the reactivity and equality of the opening and closing of the pupils in response to light. When a bright light shines into each eye, both pupils become small; with the bright light taken away (in a dimly lit room) both pupils become larger. A pupil that doesn't react to light, or pupils that are clearly unequal, usually means very serious and often life-threatening brain disease. Eyes are a mirror of the brain in another way: with a fine-beamed light and a magnifying glass (an instrument called an ophthalmoscope) one can see the blood vessels and optic nerve-head at the back of the eyeball and can estimate the pressure in the fluid-system of the brain. When central nervous system pressure is increased, especially past the age of two, when the bones have grown together so that the boney bowl that holds the brain cannot expand, the brain can be seriously threatened by squeezing. Finally, looking at the blood vessels at the back of the eyeball (with the ophthalmoscope) one gets to look directly at the body's blood-vascular system and assess the healthiness of its condition.

The white part of the eye is covered with a thin membrane called conjunctiva; this membrane (like all living tissue) is crisscrossed by tiny blood vessels. These tiny vessels can become engorged in response to inflammation (such as an allergic reaction) or to infection (such as viral or bacterial conjunctivitis) giving a condition called "pink-eye."

The eyes are naturally washed by tears. Tears are made in the lacrimal glands, small structures at the outer corners of the upper lids. Tears wash from the outer corners of the eyes to the inner corners, where they drain through the tear ducts into the nose — which is why we get a runny nose when we cry. Often in young babies the tear ducts are partially blocked, so that they have a continual drying of tears and matter at the inner corners of their eyes.

The skin around the eyes is very loose and will swell with fluid easily. Eyes get puffy-looking from crying, from an allergic reaction in or around the eyes, from insect bites near the eyes, and from other general body conditions that cause the body to retain fluids.

The hair follicles on the eyelids share the same conditions found in other hair follicles: seborrhea, breakage, and infection with parasites. In addition they sometimes become infected with tiny abscesses.

Babies are relatively farsighted and see better at some distance. This is why you may notice your baby staring with more fascination at the kitchen curtains, a few feet away, than at your own nearby face. This farsightedness diminishes as the child grows. By 4 months a child should be noticing most things in his/her world, with eyes that work well together to follow movement. Sometimes, with fatigue, one eye will appear to drift inward or outward; if this persists to the age of 6 months the child's eyes should be examined professionally, for it can mean an imbalance of the muscles that move the eyes and the child may need some special exercises or other helps to overcome the condition and retain an acute eyesight that coordinates both eyes together. By 5 years a child should be able to see billboards at a distance; many nearsighted children are never aware, until they are fitted with glasses, that most of us can see the separate leaves on trees and the separate stones on a gravel path.

Children in school should be able to see what is on the blackboard even when they are at the far end of the classroom. Most schools perform yearly eye examinations for children. If this examination suggests that your child has a visual problem, the child should be checked by a specialist. Even if your child has passed the school eye examination, if s/he complains of headaches after close work or of not being able to see well, it is a good idea to have the eyes checked by an ophthalmologist, for there are subtle vision problems (like astigmatism, in which the visual picture is irregularly distorted) that cause eye strain but may not be picked up by the visual screen at school.

Nose. Little babies breathe through their noses. They learn later how to breathe through their mouths. When they have a cold or are otherwise stuffed up they can become quite restless and fussy if they are not yet skillful in mouth-breathing.

Allergies often affect the blood vessels in the inner mucous membranes of the nose, causing congestion and perhaps some clear, watery drainage. Chronically allergic children sometimes have an habitual gesture called "the allergic salute," wiping the nose with the back of the hand. This problem is not a sickness unless it causes significant distress (like crankiness), dysfunction (like restless, disturbed sleep), disability (like poor schoolwork from decreased hearing acuity), or disfigurement.

*Ears.* The external shell of the ear, the pinna, is shaped to channel sound into the ear canal. Plastic surgeons are adept at changing the shape of the ears. There are usually only cosmetic reasons for this surgery, however, and I believe that almost all purely cosmetic operations should be postponed until the child is an adolescent and old enough to decide whether the possibility of a more pleasing appearance will be worth the risks and pain associated with the surgery.

The eardrum at the back of the canal is the first place that sound hits on its way to be heard. The eardrum must be intact and elastic for hearing to be acute. The drum should appear pink and translucent, and the landmarks of the tiny bones that lie just behind the eardrum should be clear. If the drum is red, bulging, or white and thick-appearing, or if the bony landmarks are not clear, then there is probably some trouble in the middle-ear space behind the eardrum.

The middle ear is the place where the next event of hearing takes place: the sound is transmitted by the drum (or tympanic membrane) to a series of three small bones, which ultimately translate the sounds to the very small hairs that are the endings of the hearing nerve that go into the brain.

The middle ear is connected to the throat by a narrow tube called the Eustachian canal. While in adults the Eustachian canal is bent at an angle, it is relatively straight in preadolescent children. The straightness of the tube means that germs — which are always found in the mouth and throat — can more easily pass up into the middle ear space. When there is some inflammation and congestion around the opening of the tube, as with a cold or an allergic condition or even just teething, the germs can easily become locked into the middle-ear space, where they can fester and cause an infection. This is why small children are so prone to middle-ear infections, also called otitis media. Some are more prone than others; this tendency seems to run in families and probably has to do with the anatomic configuration of the middle ear, the Eustachian canal, and the throat.

An otoscope is used to examine the inner portions of the ear. Such an instrument costs about $45 and can be obtained from any medical supply house. Almost certainly an otoscope should be shared by several families. An otoscope handle can be attached to an ophthalmoscope head, a system of light and lenses for looking at the back of the eyeball. Generally, however, the use of the ophthalmoscope is complex, and the information gained is so specialized that this relatively expensive piece of equipment is not very useful in common child-health situations.

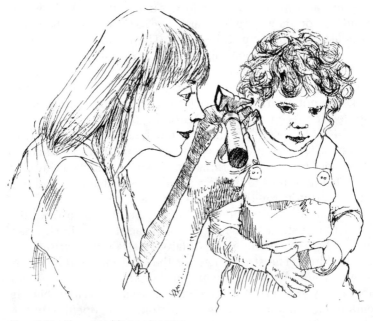

Examining the ear with an otoscope

With an otoscope and with some familiarity with the appearance of normal eardrums, you can see:

- The signs of an acute middle-ear infection: redness and, often, a bulging outward of the drum so that the usual landmarks of the little bones behind the drum are obscured.

- The signs of middle-ear fluid, which occurs in chronic middle-ear congestion (as when a child has one ear infection after another, or sometimes with chronic allergic stuffiness that impairs a child's hearing): an eardrum looks pale and dull, with the boney landmarks sometimes obscured. If your otoscope has an air bulb and you squeeze a puff of air up against the drum, it will often not move (as much as it does normally) when there is fluid behind the drum.

- A rupture of the eardrum, which can occur with trauma (when a child sticks an object into the ear canal, or sometimes with a sharp blow to the side of the head) or with a middle-ear infection: you will see a small tear in the drum, sometimes with blood or fluid leaking out of the tear. (If there is so much fluid leaking out that you cannot see the eardrum, assume there is a tear. However, do not put anything into the ear canal to clean out the fluid lest you introduce bacteria into the middle ear, which, with a tear in the drum, is exposed to outside germs.) A tear in the eardrum of a child should mend itself (with no special treatment except overcoming the middle-ear infection, if that is the reason for the tear) in a week or two. You should check the child's ear at one week after you see the tear, and again a week after that.

To look into the ear canal of an infant, pull the pinna of the ear downward in order to straighten the canal; to look in the canal of an older child pull the pinna backward and upward. If there is so much wax that you cannot see the canal (and if you are sure that there is no tear in the eardrum — that is, there has not been a recent middle-ear infection, a sharp blow to the ear, or an accident with something inserted into the ear), the wax may be cleaned out with a hydrogen-peroxide solution.

To clean the ear dilute hydrogen peroxide half and half with water and put two or three drops into the child's ear; encourage the child to lie on one side for as long as possible. If this is repeated six or eight times, over one or several days, the wax will dissolve and run out. Accumulated ear wax is not a health problem unless it makes it impossible to examine the child's eardrum or is so impacted that it impairs the child's hearing. The grandmotherly old advice is still good: never put anything into your ear that is smaller than your elbow!

With an otoscope you can also examine the ear canal, looking for scratches (after something has been put into the ear) and for redness with an accumulation of white material (external otitis), which is usually caused by "swimmer's ear," a mild infection of fungus and bacteria that children can easily get when they have been immersing their heads in used or unclean water.

Children are usually apprehensive about having their ears examined until they are used to it and know that it will not hurt. Always assume that the ear is tender — although usually it will not be. Move the pinna very gently and insert the otoscope very gently. Let the child look into your ears first.

Hearing should be acute for infants from the time of birth, with the baby noting and reacting to all kinds of sounds. Even in infancy a child's hearing can be tested accurately and painlessly by electronic equipment. For very young children hearing tests must be specially designed, but they can be given accurately and easily to children of all ages. Hearing screens in school are accurate if done conscientiously and carefully.

It is important for parents to remember to question children's hearing. If you go to a clinic and express some question about whether a child can hear well, that child can then be tested. Hearing can be difficult to assess at home for preschool and school-aged children, for they often practice a kind of selective inattention — they hear what they want to hear, and don't hear "Have you cleaned up your room?" Children who don't hear well often become very expert at lipreading. If you want to check your child's hearing at home, speak softly to the child from a place where s/he cannot read your lips, and ask a question that the child will want to hear, like, "Do you want an ice-cream cone?" Other hints about poor hearing are given by children who speak very loudly themselves and want the TV or radio turned on very loud. A preverbal child whose speech seems to be delayed, or who doesn't coo and babble very much, may have diminished hearing. Hearing problems have significant effects on children's learning, and should be corrected promptly if they are disabling.

*Mouth-throat.* Tongues can have a variety of shapes and surfaces. An odd-looking tongue is probably never the single indicator of a nutritional lack, but when it is coupled with other difficulties it may be a clue to poor nutrition. Tongue-tie — when the tongue is attached to the floor of the mouth by a short tie or frenulum — was once an explanation for a lack of speech clarity. It is now thought that if a tongue is mobile enough for a baby to nurse her/his milk from breast or bottle, then it is mobile enough for normal speech. Tongue-tie surgery is now almost obsolete.

Teeth can reflect not only health and nutrition at the time when the substance of the teeth was forming, but also general health and local care to the teeth since their eruption. The first teeth are formed while the baby is still in the womb; the second (permanent) teeth continue to be formed until about age 25. Some drugs — notably an antibiotic called tetracycline — can cause the surface enamel of the teeth to be mottled and discolored if the drug is taken while the teeth are forming; probably other chemicals have this effect as well. Severe poisoning with lead or other heavy metals sometimes causes a black line at the juncture of the teeth and the gums. If a child has fallen and hit a baby tooth so sharply that it is now dead (appearing very discolored) it usually needs no remedy. As long as it will stay in the mouth it will keep the space open for the permanent tooth that will come later.

The mucous membranes that line the mouth become pale when the body is low in iron, or anemic. One specific kind of sick-proneness that plagues some children — a trouble that is often outgrown at adolescence — is a tendency to mouth ulcers with viral infections. Small open sores on the tongue, the roof of the mouth, and elsewhere inside the mouth appear just before or during other signs of viral infection, and have a main effect of making it difficult for the child to eat and drink.

Some children can open their mouths widely enough so that the back of the throat and the tonsils can easily be seen. Others cannot open so widely. In either case the back of the tongue must be lowered so that you have a clear view. To examine a child's throat, find a good light — bright daylight, a strong lamp, or a sharply focused flashlight. Ask the child to open as widely as possible, to stick the tongue out as far as

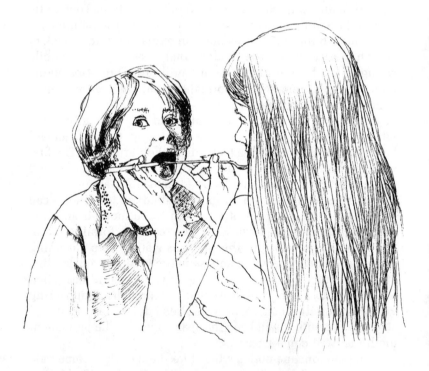

Examining the throat with a spoon handle and flashlight

possible, and to say "Aaah" — which makes the back of the tongue go down. If you cannot get a clear view of the back of the throat this way then you will need to look in a different way, using some object to depress the back of the tongue.

Few enjoy having their tongues depressed with a throat stick or spoon handle. Unless you *know* that your child will be cooperative, you should not attempt to do this with the child sitting or standing. Any flat surface will do to lie on — a bed, a table, or the floor. Have a good light source over your shoulder, or a bright and focused flashlight. Restrain the child's hands — or, if the child is old enough, have the child lie on his/her hands. It may be an almost irresistible impulse for the child to grab at the spoon. This can make the whole process even more uncomfortable. For a younger child who is thrashing and protesting, it is well to restrain the head — with another pair of hands, if you have help, or by resting your own two hands on either side of the child's jaw.

A word here about examining a protesting child. The older the child and the more experienced with examinations, the more likely the child will be to listen to reason and to cooperate. On the other hand, toddlers can rarely be convinced with words that what is happening is pleasant, or that they have any reason to allow themselves to be examined. Children who feel ill and cranky may be less cooperative than under other circumstances. There are times, then, when it will be necessary to examine a child who does not wish to be examined.

There are not many parts of the examination that are uncomfortable. Experience with health assessments — which can easily seem like a game to the child, and which do not (in the home situation) have to be completed at any particular time — will let the child know that most parts of the physical examination are not uncomfortable, embarrassing, or painful. Having done health assessments, you can convincingly remind your child that most of what you need to do when the child is ill is already easy and familiar.

Throat examinations are uncomfortable for all of us who cannot open our mouths widely and thus stay in control of the situation. The sensation of gagging — especially because it is being produced by someone else — is intensely uncomfortable; some even wonder each time if they may not vomit. This part of the examination is best left until the last if you know that your child will be upset by it. And it is best done swiftly, since anticipating discomfort can be at least as uncomfortable as the discomfort itself. If you know that your child is going to protest and be upset, then get yourself ready without fanfare and *do it*. Decide where is the best place, find the light and the spoon, get enough people to hold the child. Just before you start, tell the child what you are going to do (don't ask), remind the child that you have done it before and it is uncomfortable but won't really hurt, and that you will do it as quickly as possible. It is not pleasant to have to offend a child's dignity and autonomy by this sort of attack. If it must be done, then we can at least do it with as much grace and consideration as possible. I urge children to scream as much as they want, to try to hold still, and to be as angry at me as they need to be. I also praise lavishly (but do not reward, since this is expected good behavior) anything I can find to praise, such as good loud screaming and reasonably good holding still.

The tonsils are irregular masses on either side of the back of the throat, just above the base of the tongue. They are relatively small in early childhood, get quite large from about three until adolescence (during the time when the child is meeting and coping with most of the common respiratory infections of his/her community), and then usually shrink down to a small size during adolescence. In health they are pink and may have white material lodged in their crevices. A throat infection always means tonsillitis — inflamation of the tonsils — unless the tonsils have been removed surgically. When there is a throat infection, the tonsils either take on a lacey network of reddened blood vessels, or they become somewhat larger than usual and red all over. They may also accumulate shaggy white material on the surface, which is called exudate.

Tonsils are part of the body's defense system; antibodies are made there to combat viral and bacterial infections. Enlargement means that the tonsils are working hard. Tonsils can become so large that they appear to meet in the middle. This is good, not bad, for it means that the child's body is working hard to build immunity. It would be most unusual for a child to have difficulty swallowing or eating because the tonsils were too large. Redness and white patches — an appearance different from that when the child is in good health — may signal a throat inflammation. As with other parts of the body, you need to know what the tonsils look like when the child is well in order to be able to recognize the changes brought on by an illness.

Most throat inflammations are caused by viral infections and will not respond to any specific treatment — they are in the category of disease that we heal for ourselves. Throat infections caused by some bacteria can be treated and cured by antibiotic. To discover whether one has a strep throat (or strep tonsillitis) it is necessary to do a throat culture (see ●Throat culture — in this chapter). One cannot identify this specific infection simply by the appearance of the throat.

*Neck.* There are lymph nodes, which are structures related to the tonsils, in several places in the neck. They can become enlarged and even tender whenever they are combating a viral infection (usually a bloodstream infection) or a bacterial infection (usually confined to a specific area). Thus, the nodes located at the base of the skull in the back of the neck may be enlarged with viral infections like German measles and baby measles, or they may be enlarged when there is inflammation or infection surrounding insect bites in the scalp. Ear and throat infections often cause the lymph nodes along the side of the neck to be enlarged. Mononucleosis (which is a viral infection) and leukemia (which is a kind of malignant cancer of the blood-forming organs) cause enlargements of lymph nodes in the neck and elsewhere in the body. Large nodes may or may not be tender; once they are enlarged (which usually means that they are working hard to combat an infection), it takes several weeks — sometimes two months — for them to resume normal size.

A baby's neck is very short, and the skin of the neck is usually partly buried in folds. This means that rashes in this area can be hard to heal since exposure to light and air are important for healthy skin. The baby's neck will not lengthen to adult proportions until the child is 3 or 4.

The neck has a range of motion — forward, backward, and to each side. Limitations in that range of motion can mean muscle spasm or strain as the result of an injury. Limitation in flexing the neck forward, especially when there are other signs of illness like fever and irritability, can be an ominous sign of meningitis, an inflammation of the covering of the brain.

The thyroid gland is made up of two small bean-shaped parts on either side of the windpipe, connected across the midline by a thin strand of tissue. This gland makes a very important hormone that regulates many steps in our energy metabolism and affects our health and well-being in different ways. It can rarely be felt distinctly in children, but one should always try to feel it because any enlargement is likely to be significant. One feels for this gland by placing the thumb gently on one side of the windpipe and the first and second fingers loosely on the other side of the windpipe and waiting for the child to swallow; if there is an enlargement the gland will be felt as it bobs up and down with the swallow. If the gland is much enlarged, you will be able to see the swelling.

*The chest.* The chest should be symmetrical — or as symmetrical as any of us are in our two halves. Any marked differences in shoulder height or the shape of the curve of the ribs might lead, with further growth, to a one-sided limitation of full expansion of the lungs. The breast bone, which runs down the middle of the front of the chest, is sometimes caved in or caved outward — usually neither of these conditions leads to any serious problems with breathing. Both sides of the chest should expand and fall back even with breathing; if this does not happen — as, for instance, after an accident in which the chest has been injured — this is a serious problem.

There are lymph nodes, which drain the arms, found in the armpits. The armpit space is shaped like a square box, and one should be able to feel all of its sides.

A newborn baby's breasts are often enlarged as a result of

hormones that the baby has received from its mother; a new-born's breasts may even leak a little milk. This will all go away in a few days or weeks.

It is not uncommon for a girl (or a boy) to begin to develop in one breast before the other, early in adolescence. The swelling of the boy's breast or breasts is simply the result of the rapid hormone shifts of adolescence and will soon go away. The girl's other breast should catch up with the first in a matter of a few weeks. A rapidly growing breast may feel tight or sore. Breast development is one of the first events in a girl's adolescent development. The typical growth spurt — period of rapid growth in height and reshaping of the body from a childish to a womanly configuration — may follow soon after the beginning of breast budding or may wait for several months or even more than a year.

You can tell much about your child's breathing by observation and listening. You should know the usual rate of breathing for your child — it will vary according to age. Breathing is more rapid after exertion, when there is fever, in some kinds of poisoning (when the lungs are working to get rid of some of the poison), and when there is a respiratory infection.

If there is difficulty breathing, you should watch carefully to see whether the difficulty is with breathing in (which is called croup) or with breathing out (which is called asthma). Croup is often accompanied by a loud noise with each inspiration. Asthma may also cause noisy breathing, but with a sound at each expiration.

These distinctions can be made with the naked ear. With a stethoscope you can hear the breathing pattern more clearly. The best place for the stethoscope is on either side of the backbone about midway up the chest. When using the stethoscope the room should be very quiet. Breathing will be easier to hear if the child's mouth is open and deep, easy breaths are taken, in and out. As always, you must know what your child's breathing sounds like when s/he is well in order to understand what you hear when s/he is ill.

Examination of the heart is not a particularly important part of home health care for children. A loud heart murmur (which usually means serious heart disease) can be heard with your ear against the child's chest. Understanding the variations in the heart rate and rhythm and the sounds it makes while pumping blood requires not only the professional's experienced ear, but often a battery of machines to take pictures of the heart and its action and to measure the electrical currents of the beating heart. On the other hand, every child past 3 years of age should be able to listen to his or her heart with a stethoscope and understand that that pump brings life's blood to every part of the body, for nourishment and to cleanse the body of wastes. When you listen to the heart, the child's mouth should be closed for quiet breathing.

*The belly.* The belly contains many organs. In order to be able to think about belly pains, and to understand what you feel when you examine the belly, it is good to have some idea as to the location of these organs.

In the upper right quarter or quadrant, up under the ribs and lying just beneath the diaphragm, is the liver. Usually no more than the edge of the liver can be felt, moving up and down with breathing. The liver should not be tender. The gall bladder lies next to the liver.

In the upper left quadrant, as high up as the liver, is the spleen, an organ related to the lymph nodes in its capacity to make infection-fighting substances. It is usually felt only when there is some relatively serious illness.

In the back on either side of the backbone, near the diaphragm, are the kidneys. A newborn's kidneys are somewhat lower than at older ages. If there is infection in a kidney, tenderness is sometimes felt when a gentle punch is given at the angle of the backbone and the bottom rib.

In the lower midsection, just above the pubic bone, is the urinary bladder. When the bladder is very full of urine, an area of dullness can be tapped out (by placing the fingers of one hand firmly over that place and tapping on them with the fingers of the other hand); when there is inflammation in the bladder this tapping often causes discomfort.

Between the bladder and the kidneys are the ureters —

narrow tubes that carry the urine from the kidneys, where it is filtered out of the blood, to the bladder, where it collects until the sensation of stretch tells us that it is time to void. Pain along these tubes can be from infection or from the passage of a stone.

In the upper midsection, just under the ribs and slightly to the left, is the pancreas, an organ that makes digestive juices as well as insulin. The pancreas lies toward the back; tenderness can be elicited with deep pushing. In the center of the upper midsection are the lower esophagus, the stomach, and the upper intestine. Any or all of these can be irritated, painful, and tender from an excess of stomach juices, which are very acidic.

Coiled everywhere in the belly are the many feet of small intestine, running from the stomach to the large intestine, or colon. The muscular workings of the intestine can be heard with a stethoscope as bubbly crackles of sound, occurring at brief and regular intervals. When these sounds cannot be heard, there may be an obstruction somewhere in the digestive tract. When these sounds are louder than usual and occur in prolonged rushes separated by silence there may be overactive muscular movements, either from a hyperactive gut (as in diarrhea) or from efforts to overcome an obstruction.

In the right lower quadrant is the appendix. It is at the third point of a triangle that also includes the belly button and the crest of the hipbone. The appendix is a fingerlike projection at the joining of the small and the large intestine.

Arching in the shape of a croquet wicket, from the right lower quadrant up to the diaphragm, across the upper part of the belly and down again on the left side, is the large intestine, or colon. Here the wastes of our food are stored and excess water is absorbed in preparation for elimination of stool. When there is constipation of a significant degree one can feel hard masses, especially along the left side.

In females, the uterus lies just behind the urinary bladder. The ovaries, connected to the uterus by tubes, lie one in each lower quadrant.

The belly is best examined with a warm hand, beginning

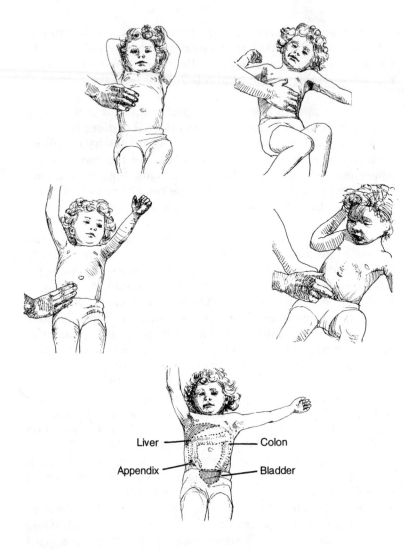

Feeling for the edge of the liver in the right upper quadrant of the belly
Feeling for the spleen in the left upper quadrant
Checking for the pain of appendicitis in the right lower quadrant
Tapping over the bladder: tenderness here might mean a urinary tract infection
Diagram showing some of the organs in the belly

with a very gentle touch and gradually pressing in the various areas with a firmer touch. The child should be lying on his/her back with knees bent and hands at the sides for the greatest relaxation of the superificial muscles of the belly. Taking very deep breaths also helps to relax muscles and distracts the child from the sensation of tickling. As with every part of the examination, if you know your child well and have felt the belly often, you will be able to notice when there are changes.

When I was a medical student and my first child was nearly five, he complained so severely about a belly ache that I was worried he might have appendicitis. I asked him to lie down on his bed and sat beside him to examine his belly. As I laid my hand on him to begin to press, he screamed with pain. I asked him if his belly were really that tender and he said, with tears in his eyes, "No, no, you're sitting on my foot!" Be sure to talk to your child while you are examining, asking how it feels, where it hurts, and what kind of pain or tenderness is being experienced.

*Girls' genitals.* It is interesting that in our efforts to give children the names for those parts of their bodies that have been considered secret, shameful, and nameless, we have tended, for girls, to assign names wrongly. The one word that mothers and young girls are likely to know for the whole external genital area is the vagina. The vagina is only the tube that connects the external genital structures to the cervix, the opening of the uterus. The general term for the layers and folds of the external genitals is vulva. While preadolescent girls rarely have vaginal problems, vulvar irritations and inflammations are fairly common. The other specific part that a child should be able to name, because it is sensitive and reactive to touch, is the clitoris.

At some point in the growing-up years girls, like boys, may ask their mothers not to examine their genitals. As this time approaches girls should be shown how, and then urged, to examine themselves with a mirror. Mothers, of course, should also examine themselves (with a mirror) in the genital area, to be familiar with the genital anatomy of daughters.

Rarely, a girl may have a hernia that extends into the vulva. A piece of small intestine can slide out of the belly cavity, through a small space (the inguinal ring, located in the groin), and down into or just above the external vulvar fold. The hernia causes swelling in this area, and sometimes tenderness.

*Boys' genitals.* There are no absolute health reasons for the circumcision of boys. The social situation within the family — for instance, if the boy's father has been circumcised — may be a valid reason for a circumcision. Circumcised or not, boys need to be taught about genital cleanliness. A short circumcision leaves the sensitive glans — the tip of the penis — exposed and subject to irritation. Boys who are not circumcised, or who have a long cuff of foreskin after a circumcision, can develop irritations under the foreskin. This cuff must be pulled back for thorough cleansing at bath time, at first by the adult who bathes the child and later by the child himself.

Both testes should be felt as firm little beans in either side of the sac of the scrotum. These little organs are pulled up into the body when the air temperature is cold, so after a warm bath is usually the best time to check for the testes. Before birth — and sometimes for a period after birth — the testes are still in the abdominal cavity. They must migrate down into the scrotum before adolescence and the beginning of formation of sperm, because sperm cannot be made at the warm temperature inside the belly. Once both testes have been felt in the scrotum, you will know that the migration has been completed.

Boys have hernias at the inguinal area more often than girls do. A boy's hernia slides down into the scrotum and appears as a suddenly enlarged and usually one-sided swelling. Other causes of swelling in the scrotum are due to inflammation or injury — both cause tenderness, usually more tenderness than is caused by a hernia.

*The legs and feet.* Many of us do not have perfectly straight legs and feet. Knock-knees, bowlegs, flat feet, and feet that are turned in or out may run in families. They are usually correctible only with major orthopedic care, often involving surgery. The first rule to consider in the evaluation of leg and foot problems is to watch the child at play and decide whether s/he is significantly slower or more clumsy than age mates. Occasionally the child will complain of pain or appear to have less staying power in vigorous exercise than you would expect. If the child is hampered in any of these ways, then you will want to have an orthopedist evaluate the situation and outline the steps for making corrections. You and the child can then decide whether those repairs are desired. In the absence of distress, disability, or dysfunction, there is probably no reason for urgency in these matters. Problems of disfigurement should wait (unless for technical reasons correction must be done at an early age) until the child is old enough to make an informed decision about whether the risks and costs of correction are outweighed by the value of altering the disfigurement.

The back. The spine is sometimes not straight but shows an S-shaped curve. This scoliosis can be observed by having the child bend forward, head flopped loosely down and arms hung at ease, like Raggedy Ann. Trace the spinal column with your finger, to be sure it is straight. Note whether the lower ribs and the crests of the hipbones on each side are at the same height, each with its pair. Imaginary lines connecting the ribs and the hipbones should be perpendicular to the line of the spinal column. This examination must be done once each year, for a previously straight spine can develop a curve as it grows.

The significance of this part of the examination is that a scoliosis can quickly become exaggerated in its curvature at the time of the adolescent growth spurt. A marked curve can cause a hunchbacked appearance and a breathing impairment if one side of the ribcage is compressed. A spinal curvature should be professionally evaluated before the growth spurt begins.

The skin and nails. Skin varies tremendously in color (caused by different amounts of dark pigment in cells below the surface), and in texture, dryness, and elasticity. It also

varies in its tendency to become infected and in the rapidity
of its self-healing. Skin is our protection against invasion by
the foreign world that surrounds us. Any break — a scrape, a
burn, or a cut — makes us vulnerable to infection.

Children's skin heals much more rapidly than adults' skin,
often requiring no more than exposure to air and light to repair
itself. Rashes and other kinds of breaks in the integrity of the
skin covering should be observed for reddening where the
break is, reddening in the surrounding skin area, weeping clear
fluid, oozing yellow creamy material or blood, and a raised
and bumpy or smooth feel. It is also important to note whether
the changes are spreading out from a central area or appearing
separately and distinctly on other parts of the body.

Certain skin changes suggest dietary deficiencies. These
include a decrease in elasticity, an increase in dryness, and a
tendency to become rashy or to heal slowly. Nails also reflect
nutrition; nails that have become ridged, mottled, discolored,
or very breakable may indicate an inadequate diet. Remember
that learning what the correct diet is for any individual is a
matter of trial and error, for we all have slightly different
nutritional needs.

*The nervous system.* The best examination you can make
of the functioning of your child's nervous system is to observe
the child closely in play and other daily activities. Changes in
balance and coordination, in clumsiness (falling and bumping
into things), and in the ability to be aware of what is going on
in the immediate environment, can be of significant importance in reflecting the function of the nervous system.

*Tests.* As part of the physical examination, mothers can
also learn to perform some simple tests at home.
* Urine tests. An informative test of urine can be done at
  home with the use of a prepared dipstick. The child voids
  a little urine into a clean but not sterile cup. Dip the small
  plastic strip into the urine, hold the bottle sideways so
  that you can compare the colors on the dipstick with the
  sample colors printed on the bottle, and use a watch with

a sweep-second hand. The instructions on the bottle tell you how long after dipping you should note the color changes in the four areas of the dipstick that measure the presence of different substances in the urine.

Protein should not be present in the urine, except occasionally in trace amounts when the child has not bathed for some time. Protein in the urine suggests a malfunction of the kidneys.

Sugar should not be present in the urine, although occasionally it will appear in a single voiding after the child has eaten a large amount of sweet food at one time.

Ketones should not be present in the urine. If sugar is present, with or without the presence of ketones, this suggests diabetes. If ketones alone are present, this suggests that the child has not had very much to eat and is reflecting a metabolic change associated with short-term starvation. One sees ketones, for instance, after a child has been vomiting, or after a period of not eating. The presence of ketones is not alarming but it is an indicator of the severity of an illness.

Blood should not be in the urine, although it will appear when the child's urethral sphincter (the opening for urine on the tip of the penis or inside the folds of the vulva) is red, raw, and irritated, and when an adolescent is menstruating. In some individuals, blood appears in urine regularly after vigorous exercise. If blood appears in urine from the bladder, this suggests a urine infection or a malfunction of the kidneys.

The dipstick also measures pH (acidity) of urine; this information is of no particular use in a routine urine check, but is useful when the child is using some medications recommended for treating urine infections.

Except for ketones, when you know that the child has not been able to eat, presence of these substances in the urine is reason to consult a professional.

The dipsticks are called Labstix and are manufactured by the Ames Company in Elkhart, Indiana. They can be purchased through any pharmacist without a prescription.

A bottle of 100 costs less than $20; this is the sort of purchase that could be shared by a group of households.

Some children are known to be prone to urinary-tract infections. Urine infections are not uncommon, especially in females. They can cause acute illness with high fever and vomiting, or a mild illness that is less dramatic. There are no regular symptoms or signs of a urinary-tract infection, and to be sure of the diagnosis you must examine the urine to see if it contains bacteria.

A kit called Uricult can be used to check a urine culture — a test for bacteria — at home. A sample of the child's urine is collected after carefully washing the urethral sphincter with pHisohex or Betadyne soap and rinsing well with clean water. You need only a few drops of urine for the test. If possible you should collect urine from the middle of the stream, as the first few drops may contain bacteria that has washed off the child's skin. A sterile cup is supplied with the kit.

A coated dipstick is inserted in the urine, then placed in a small container. This container is kept in the oven, pilot light on; the temperature should be 37.2° C/99° F, which you can check with a thermometer.

The kit comes with instructions for interpreting the test; it can be read after 18–24 hours of incubation. In this as in all tests that you might do at home, you should ask for instruction and help from a medical professional until you feel confident in doing the test.

In a child with recurrent urine infections, you and the doctor can work out a system to arrange to start appropriate treatment. (Children with urine infections should be tested to determine whether the cause of the infections is a treatable anatomic anomaly.) The urine should be cultured again four days after starting treatment to be sure that the treatment has cleansed the urine of bacteria. An equally important value in doing this test at home is to assure yourself that a child with an undefined illness does not have a urine infection.

The Uricult kit can be purchased at a medical-surgical

supply house. They are supplied in boxes of 10 for a cost of less than $10.

• Hematocrit. Each year when you give your child a physical examination, you will want to do a blood test to find out how much hemoglobin (the iron-containing substance that carries oxygen) is in the blood. Measuring hemoglobin is a moderately complicated laboratory test, but we get a rough but fairly accurate estimate of the amount of hemo-globin by a test of the hematocrit, a very simple measurement.

The hematocrit is measured by finding out what pro-portion of the blood is cells (formed elements) and what proportion is the watery part. This is because a large part of the red cells in the blood is hemoglobin, and because most of the cells in the blood are red cells. We know from experience what proportion of the blood of adult women and men and what proportion of the blood of babies and young children will be cells, as opposed to the watery part, when there is no anemia. If a tiny tube of blood is spun around and around in a centrifuge (a small machine with a motor that spins a drum around, rather like the spin cycle in an automatic washing machine) the cells will settle at one end of the tube because they are heavier than the watery part, which stays at the other end of the tube.

To measure the hematocrit, clean the fleshy part of a fingertip with an alcohol swab and then prick the finger with a small, sharp metal knife called a lancet, which is packaged in an individual sterile package. The lancet is made so it can only go into the finger so far and no farther. Wipe off the first drop of blood that appears with a dry, sterile sponge (the first drop is often diluted with the alcohol that we used to clean the finger) and then hold the end of a tiny glass tube to the drop of blood that comes out of the little cut. The tube will fill with blood (by "capillary action") while it is in contact with the drop of blood. There is a line near the top of the tube that shows how far to fill the tube. Always fill two tubes for each measurement to give a check on accuracy. When each tube

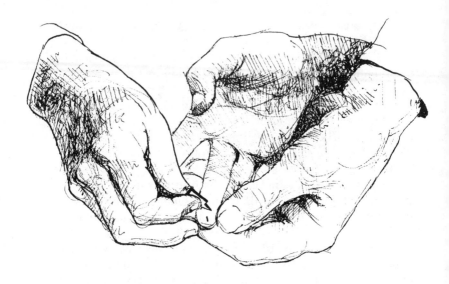

A finger prick with a lancet. The blood is used to measure the hematocrit, a test for anemia.

is filled with blood to the line, the other end is stuck into a small tray of special soft clay; a tiny plug of this clay stays in the tube and keeps the blood from coming out of the tube when it is spun around. The tubes are fitted into the slots of the centrifuge (with the clay plug toward the outside rim of the machine) and the centrifuge is run. When it stops, the proportion of cells (the line where the red material at one end of the tube is separated from the clear or white material at the other end of the tube) is measured on a special ruler that is provided with the centrifuge.

Lancets, swabs, and glass tubes cost pennies. A centrifuge costs about $300, can be bought at a medical-surgical supply house, and should certainly be shared by many families.

If the hematocrit reading is below normal for a person's age and sex, there is anemia. That anemia might be due to a variety of causes. The hematocrit for children 6 and older should be at least 34 percent; for children 4 months to 6 years it should be at least 32 percent. With a hematocrit of 28 percent or less one should have laboratory tests to determine the cause before any treatment is begun.

• Throat culture. When your child has a sore throat, you may want to take a throat culture to see if he has strep sore throat or strep tonsillitis.

Some states have a free throat-culture program. Ask your doctor how you might do throat cultures at home. You will need the same equipment and procedures as for a throat examination, and also a sterile swab and a "carrying medium," a material to keep the bacteria alive during transport to a laboratory. There are always bacteria in the human throat; the question when taking a culture is to discover which specific bacteria are growing there. Each of the two tonsils must be firmly scrubbed with the sterile swab. The swab is then put into the carrying medium — usually either a packet of salt crystals or a liquid broth in a tube — and mailed or brought to a laboratory. Alternatively, you can smear the swab on a culture plate and incubate it overnight in a gas oven with the pilot on. If your state does not have a free program of incubating and interpreting throat cultures, perhaps your neighborhood clinic will sell culture plates to you and teach you the simple techniques of incubation and interpretation.

All parts of the physical examination require two things of you: the practice of some fairly simple skills, and repeated, considered, and attentive focusing on your child. The skills can be practiced on yourself, other mothers and their children, and on any child who will play with you as your subject. Practice and practice until you feel confident of your eyes and hands and ears.

Knowing your own child, in the matter of health assessments, means for the most part an organizing of what you already know as the child's mother. You have looked and listened and felt every day in the course of your ordinary caretaking. Doing a formal health assessment gives you an opportunity to pull together what you already know.

Each of us is different from every other. Knowing one person very well — yourself, or your child — enables you to recognize changes as they occur. As a mother you are thus in a better position than a doctor to notice changes — even though you will often want professional help in interpreting those changes. If you have more than one child — or take care of children other than your own — you will learn some of the range of expected variations among children. A doctor can never know your child as well as you do — s/he can only use knowledge and experience based on some idea of "average" or "normal."

Most importantly, consult with your child about these examinations. Talk about the ideas and the skills, about what you are observing, and how good it is to have this kind of knowledge. These are games of understanding that delight children. As the responsibility for this knowledge is transferred to children, they will know pleasure and pride in assessing their own healthiness.

# CHAPTER 4

# Remedies — Old and New

Healing comes from within. Every culture evolves a set of remedies that are given for dis-ease: some are thought to "cure," while others comfort, take away pain, overcome dysfunction or disability, or hide or improve a disfigurement. But no remedy, in and of itself, will restore good health. One's underlying good health and wish to be well do most or all of the real healing.

There are two general classes of remedies that we need to know about and use in home health care. Some remedies involve the use of *substances* that might be given to the ill person to eat or drink, to be rubbed on the skin, used in a poultice, or dissolved in water for a bath. Other remedies involve the use of *skills* like massage, bandaging, removing foreign bodies, and the methods of preparing and giving substance remedies.

The remedies of our culture include a few really curative substances; others are being developed. There may soon be substances that help cure viral infections, for instance. But most of our remedies, including most of the manufactured chemical drugs sold only on a doctor's prescription, are not curative. They allay symptoms, they offer comfort and support, and they assure the person who is ill that s/he is being taken care of. The remedies commonly used now in the United States are not exactly the same as the remedies used in the United

Kingdom or in the USSR. At the same time, most of the remedies of these advanced countries are not so very different from
the folk remedies known and used in every culture for
centuries.

Doctors know about one group of remedies — the prescription drugs. These are remedies that have been judged to require
the supervision of a professional for their use; presumably the
sick person is at some risk of harm when using these remedies.
This risk of harm is quite often real and significant — before
anyone takes a prescription drug, or gives a prescription drug
to a child, s/he should read the package insert (or the compi-
lation of package inserts in book form, the *Physician's Desk
Reference*) and be informed about what those risks are.

Other prescription drugs are in fact relatively mild and
have few or rare side effects. No substance remedy is *entirely*
benign or has no side effects or no possibility of undesired
consequences. Penicillin, when taken by mouth, is one such
relatively benign drug.

There is, of course, a statistically rare possibility of a severe
allergic reaction to penicillin — as there is for most drugs. But
you — as the person giving penicillin to your own child —
have all of the information that must be taken into consideration before giving penicillin to the child and risking that allergic reaction. That information includes the family history of
allergies, the family history of allergy to penicillin, and the
child's own past history of allergic symptoms and drug-taking.
Aside from that statistically rare risk of drug allergy, penicillin
taken by mouth has been reported only to cause, occasionally,
the undesirable effects of nausea, vomiting, and/or diarrhea.
Used prudently by a mother, and only on occasions when
penicillin is known to be an appropriate remedy — that is,
when a culture of a throat infection or a skin infection has
demonstrated that the infection is caused by the bacteria
known as beta-hemolytic streptococcus or by some other bacteria sensitive to penicillin — this drug is efficacious, inexpensive, and relatively nonhazardous. I believe that mothers can
learn to make wise decisions about treating their children with
penicillin in many instances of childhood illness. Later in this

chapter we will consider other prescription drugs for which decisions about use might safely and sensibly be in the hands of mothers.

Doctors know somewhat less about two other broad groups of substance remedies: those manufactured drugs that the medical-pharmaceutical establishment have decided can be sold without a prescription (over-the-counter, or OTC), and those herbs and foods that have long been thought to be helpful in specific kinds of dis-ease but are not now in favor as substance remedies in the professional practice of medicine.

Other remedies are skills, ways of doing things. Doctors and nurses and other medical professionals — especially those who work in hospital emergency rooms — know many relatively simple skills that are useful in treating a variety of common childhood diseases. Other skills are less well known to professionals than they are to mothers who, through the ages, have helped their children heal themselves at home. Altogether, there is a large body of home health remedies that mothers can use wisely and skillfully.

## Effects of Remedies

Any remedy can have a variety of effects. These effects are the same whether the remedy is given by a mother (with or without the supervision of a medical professional) or by medical experts (with or without consultation with the child and her mother).

*Remedies that Strengthen.* A remedy can strengthen the ill or hurt child, so that her/his own natural defenses can most effectively overcome the causes and effects of the dis-ease. Here are some examples of remedies that strengthen:

- The reassurance that the dis-ease will end, that the child is strong, loved, and cared for, and that s/he will get better. This remedy is the single most important and universal treatment for all dis-ease.
- The offer of a variety of health-promoting foods, from which the child can make a selection.

- The provision of clean fresh air and sunshine, and some opportunity for exercise — if only relatively passive exercise in bed.
- The giving of specific strengthening substances, such as the administration of supplementary iron to an iron-deficient and anemic child.

*Remedies that treat the cause of disease.* Remedies can remove or overcome the cause of the illness, when that cause can be determined or presumed. Modern Western medicine focuses on this particular principle of treatment, and medical professionals often like to believe that this is the only or at least the most important aspect of treatment. In fact, there are relatively few instances — out of all the ills that plague us — in which we *know* with certainty the cause of the dis-ease, and have some *specific* treatment. More often we guess at the cause and treat with some nonspecific remedy, hoping that the consequences of the remedy will not be worse than the dis-ease. Most curative drugs are obtained by a doctor's prescription. Some examples of remedies that act directly on the causes of dis-ease are:

- Removing a lead-poisoned child from an environment that contains lead, or removing the lead (such as chips or dust of lead-containing paint) from the environment of the child.
- Giving a specific antibacterial drug that is known to be effective in slowing or stopping an infection by an identified microorganism. If urine (which is ordinarily sterile) is cultured and found to contain the bacteria E. *coli* — a microorganism nearly always found in human feces — a sulfa drug (such as Gantrisin) will prevent the bacteria from multiplying, while a semisynthetic penicillin (such as ampicillin) will kill the bacteria. The effects of the infection on the body, such as inflammation, are still repaired by the body's own defenses.
- Giving a specific nutrient, the lack of which causes disease. Too little calcium or vitamin D causes rickets, too little iodine results in a goiter and an insufficient produc-

tion of the thyroid hormone, too little protein causes a state of malnourishment called kwashiorkor. In each instance, the cause of the disease can be overcome by feeding increased amounts of the specific nutrient lacking.

*Remedies that treat the symptoms of dis-ease.* Remedies can be given to treat the symptoms of the illness. Symptoms can be overcome, they can be compensated for, or they can be masked. In every case we are essentially comforting the child until his/her personal (physical, psychological, and spiritual) resources can cope with the causes and effects of the dis-ease. Sometimes symptoms themselves can cause significant harm. A raging diarrhea in an infant can cause a raw rash in the diaper area. Vomiting and diarrhea can cause dehydration and a disturbance in the balance of body salts. A high fever can precipitate a seizure in a seizure-prone child. Removing or modifying symptoms, therefore, can bring a more direct benefit than just comfort. In every case, however, symptomatic treatment is a holding action until the underlying illness can be overcome by the child's own self-healing mechanisms. Here are some examples of remedies that mask, overcome, or compensate for symptoms:

- The drug theophylline can remove or lessen the symptom of asthma (wheezing) by dilating the breathing tubes, until the cause of the asthma — which might be infection, allergy, stress, or some combination of these — can be overcome.
- Baths with bicarbonate of soda or cornstarch added are soothing and decrease the itch of poison-ivy rash while the skin heals itself.
- Aspirin (or, to a lesser extent, acetoaminophen) masks the symptom of fever. As long as you give aspirin on a regular schedule of every four hours, the child will remain less warm or even fever free. This may be a comfort if the child is restless or drowsy and uncomfortable from the increased body temperature. But it is important to treat the child and not just the fever. Aspirin should not be given just to treat yourself and your own worry. A fever by itself is not

harmful if the child is not unduly uncomfortable. Fast-rising fevers (as at the beginning of an illness) and very high fevers (above 40° C/104° F) may be somewhat bothersome for the child, but a lower level of fever need not be brought to a normal temperature and may even give the child some advantage in fighting off an infection.

*Remedies that reinforce trust.* Remedies can be given to reinforce confidence in the caretaker's ability to help the child heal his/her body. One reason that self-help home health care for children has always been so effective is that the ingredient of faith or trust already exists in the enduring relationship between mother and child. "I trust you because I know, from past experience, that you care about me and will help me." This aspect of assistance in healing is always potentially present between mother and child — even when your child looks at you askance and says, in effect, "Are you *sure* this will make me better?"

"Trust me because you know, from past experience, that I am knowledgeable and competent to assist you in your healing" is a part of the mother-child relationship that can be fostered and developed. Children are cranky and irritable when they feel ill; they may protest every attempt to help. But there is, for most children, no one who has proven more often and more reliably that she knows what will help than the mother.

Many of our remedies have the reinforcing of this trust as their primary value. For anyone, child or adult, whose dis-ease is sufficient to call for help in the healing process, the fostering and strengthening of this trust is a critical and important ingredient in restoring health. Meeting the expectations or wishes of the one who is ill demonstrates that "someone really knows me well, knows what I need, and cares enough to provide it for me." Here are some examples of remedies that reinforce trust, thereby strengthening the child's own healing potential:

- Rubbing on lotions, liniments, or creams promotes healing rest, eases aches, and gives the comfort of skin-to-skin contact.
- Bringing cold drinks or hot teas provides something to do

("sip it slowly"), health-promoting nutrients, a pleasant taste, and comfort of aches, chills, or fevers.

● Giving simple medicinal remedies — that may or may not have a specific effect on symptoms or tho hoaling piocess — is reassuring and comforting. A mixture of honey and lemon juice, given in moderation, will never hurt, and encourages the child to feel that "something is being done" about a cough (honey should not be fed before 9 months; it can cause infection in infants); peppermint or camomile tea is tasty, soothing, and harmless; specially prepared "sick" foods, high in protein — chicken, fish, yogurt, or eggs, whatever the child prefers — are thoughtful reassurances that you know what will make the child better.

## Plan of Treatment

A careful plan of treatment for a child's illness will always consider these four kinds of questions:

● What safe and simple remedies can be given to strengthen the child?

● Are the child's complaints likely to be due to an illness that will respond to a curative drug? What are the risks of giving such a drug? How carefully should the decision about giving a curative remedy be made, according to the associated risks of harm from the remedy? At what point in the illness will you want to consult a professional to consider the giving of a drug that might be curative?

● What safe and simple remedies can be given to relieve the child's symptoms? Can these remedies be given before consulting a professional (if that step is contemplated) without disguising the illness?

● What safe and simple remedies can be given to reassure the child that you will guide him/her through healing to health?

The process of deciding on a treatment plan is not essentially different for a mother than for a medical professional. The story of the dis-ease is reviewed and the child is examined

carefully. An interval of time is allowed to pass in order to
learn what the course of the illness will be, unless the onset is
so abrupt and severe that initial symptoms cannot be allayed
or the child cannot be comforted. A decision is made — a
decision that may be revised several times through the course
of the illness — about the probable nature, extent, and cause
of the trouble, and treatments are chosen.

The professional has broad experience in the interpretation of the patient's story about the onset and course of the
illness, in the discovery of signs in the physical examination,
and in the use of special technical means for testing illness
effects, like laboratory tests and electrocardiographs. On the
other hand, a mother has the advantages of knowing the child's
usual healthy state and usual reactions to illness and of not
being bound by the medical professional's systematic blinders,
which may force the illness into a category where it fits only
approximately. A mother also cares, personally and intimately,
that the child regains health as smoothly and as quickly as
possible, will remain accessible to the child throughout the
entire process of healing, and is known to the child as trust-
worthy. For most childhood dis-ease, a mother can work out
an appropriate and individualized treatment plan for her child;
in some instances she will want the supervision, assistance,
and teaching of a medical professional. And there are rare
instances of severe illness or injury when a mother may wish
to give over her entire helping responsibility to a medical
professional. It is important to remember that, even so, she has
taken the responsibility of choosing a doctor and of deciding
to place the child's welfare in the doctor's hands. A mother's
responsibility for her child's welfare is profoundly binding.

### Substance Remedies

There are three general categories of substance remedies:
- Manufactured chemicals that are available only on the
  prescription of a physician.
- Manufactured chemicals that are available without a prescription, over-the-counter (OTC).

- Foods and herbs that can be bought, grown, or gathered wild and that are not ordinarily thought of as useful remedies by our medical professionals. Strictly speaking, peppermint tea bought in a health-food store is an OTC substance, but since its healing qualities are better known to mothers than to professional medical experts I will include it under *Herbal Remedies*.

There are general principles for the use of any substance remedies for children. The first is that we wish to use the mildest, least hazardous remedy that will serve the purpose. For instance, aspirin is an effective and relatively benign drug. It is, in appropriate doses, effective as a relaxant and sleep-inducer (and safer than barbiturate sleeping medicines), effective as a pain reliever (and safer than narcotics), and effective for reducing inflammation (and safer than steroid hormones). But aspirin can irritate the lining of the stomach and almost always alters the body's ability to stop bleeding efficiently. Before giving aspirin, consider:

- For relaxation and sleep: a warm bath, a drink of warm milk or camomile tea, a massage.
- For the pain of a headache: a rest in a dark room with pleasant music, a neck massage, a cold compress of witch hazel, acupressure.
- For the inflammation of swollen insect bites: a poultice of baking soda and water, followed by a dressing of aloe.

If these benign remedies are not sufficient, aspirin may be needed. But we should always begin with remedies that are gentle and soothing, are likely to be effective, and have minimal harmful side effects.

The second general principle for choosing a substance remedy is to respect the symptom. Symptoms causing distress, dysfunction, disability, and disfigurement are messages about dis-ease, and may even serve some useful purpose in the process of healing. Vomiting is the body's way of getting rid of noxious substances in the stomach. It is also a useful mechanism for a stomach that is not working well, as when a viral infection has caused some inflammation. Emptying the stomach of its contents may be necessary to allow the stomach to heal itself. Clearly, it makes no sense to give, at the first sign of vomiting, a fairly potent drug that acts on the brain — which is what most antivomiting drugs do. Only when the child is in danger of becoming exhausted or dehydrated, or the vomiting is dry and painful retching from an empty stomach, and when simple and safe remedies have been tried and have not helped, should we think about giving more potent substances.

Similarly, diarrhea may be the body's way of emptying the bowel so it can heal. A fever may strengthen the body's ability to fight off an infection. A headache may be a signal that the body needs rest and peace, a withdrawal from activities and responsibilities. *All* signs and symptoms of dis-ease should be interpreted to mean that the body is asking for some change, some respite from present stresses. One should immediately begin to think about taking first steps to strengthen and support the child's capacity for self-healing. To take direct measures to remove a symptom, such as pushing the child back into her/his busy life, is an approach that can fail to appreciate the meaning of symptoms and thus can interfere with rather than assist in healing in its broadest sense. This approach can also teach the child that the body's messages are invalid, to be attended to only as something to be gotten rid of. It is difficult to think of a dis-ease situation in which strengthening and reassurance should not be given their full due as healing measures.

A third general principle applies to all but a small group of curative substances: give only as much of a substance as seems to be needed to achieve the result desired. Every substance remedy has potential side effects. When we give substance remedies to children we run the risk of demanding that the child accept a substance that can upset the equilibrium of the body more than it assists in healing; the cure can be worse than the disease. Undesired side effects can produce new symptoms (as when an antibiotic produces diarrhea and a rash by its effect on the balance of microorganisms in the bowel) or can interfere with the body's own healing mechanisms (as when a sweet cough medicine depresses the child's appetite for strengthening foods).

The exceptions to this rule are few: some substances are known to have their desired effect only when given on a regular schedule, never missing a dose, and for a specified number of days. Most of these are prescription drugs. One example is penicillin given for a strep throat: it must be given every eight hours, on a careful schedule, and for a full ten days. Ordinarily the prescription will be written for thirty doses, and you will be told to use all that is prescribed. Another example is a cream or liquid prescribed for a monilial infection — "thrush" in a baby's mouth or a red, raised rash in the diaper area. The drug must be given for three or four days after all symptoms disappear, or the infection is likely to reappear. Whenever you are given a prescription for a substance remedy you must ask whether the drug is to be given on a very rigid schedule, never missing a dose or varying the hour, and for how many days or doses it is to be given.

The healing powers of healthy children are remarkable and must be respected. For instance, infants who lie in wet or soiled diapers, as all do, may develop quite angry-looking skin rashes in the diaper area. Creams, ointments, powders, and lotions are manufactured and recommended to treat these rashes. In fact, there is one best treatment: leave the baby's bottom exposed to air and light — as much as possible and convenient — and the skin will transform itself in a matter of hours. Unless the rash becomes infected with some bacteria or fungus (which may require an antibacterial or antifungal cream to assist in healing), the only use for substances applied to the baby's bottom is to protect or waterproof the skin from further contact with urine and feces when a child must be diapered.

We are justly called an overmedicated society, having been sold the notion that there *should be* a magic-bullet pill or drug for every ailment and dis-ease. Not every symptom will require the giving of a substance; often our self-healing potential works its effect, out of our underlying healthiness that makes up the reserve of healing, without any need or help from administered substances.

The last general principle for giving children substance remedies (except those in tablet or capsule form) is to taste or try the medicine yourself. There are two reasons for this. The first is that many substances given by mouth have distinctive or even unpleasant tastes; some ointments sting or give a warm sensation. A child can feel helpless when some unpleasant substance is applied to the skin or put into the child's mouth. The least we can do — if it is indeed necessary "for the child's own good" to give the medicine — is to know what it is that we are giving. The second reason is that errors in the compounding of substances are always possible. Children have been made ill, or even died, from herbal remedies where an error in plant identification was made. But such errors are by no means confined to substances gathered from the wild. Both OTC drugs and prescription drugs have on occasion been made in the wrong concentration or with the wrong ingredients. These accidents are, of course, quite rare, but we would be foolish to trust unquestioningly those who prepare substances for our children. Simply by trying a medicine before I give it to my child, I cannot be sure that the medicine is what it is supposed to be. But I can reassure myself in some small degree if I use it before s/he does.

Here are some examples of substance remedies that mothers can use wisely at home. This list only gives *examples* of substances that can be used at home, examples chosen to help you learn the kinds of information you need to make sensible and safe choices about giving substance remedies.

**Prescription Drugs**

By definition, prescription drugs are not available except on the order of a doctor. When you clearly understand the uses, side effects, hazards, and reasons for giving a prescription drug, you might arrange with a doctor to keep a small supply of the drug at home, or, preferably, to have the doctor agree to phone in a prescription for you whenever you and the doctor believe that use of the drug is needed. The latter plan works only when you can have immediate access to the doctor by telephone. *If you keep drugs in the house, always keep them* in a locked container. Toddlers and mischievous older children must not be allowed access to substances that can poison them. Prescription drugs should not be given to infants younger than 6 months except on the specific recommendation of a professional.

- Codeine. Codeine is a drug derived from the opium plant. It is a mild analgesic, which means that it acts to relieve pain by affecting the brain. Formerly painful sensations are no longer perceived as being so painful. It also reduces the urge to cough, again by acting on the brain. For both of these effects it is useful for children. It also has some sedative effect — tending to calm or tranquilize — but it should not ordinarily be used for this purpose for children.

  Codeine is a narcotic and should not be used unless it is really needed. But there are occasions when a child's pain is severe and you will want to have something stronger than aspirin. Codeine can then be given in addition to aspirin; that is, a half hour after you have given aspirin and have had a chance to see that the aspirin is not going to be enough to dull the pain. Some common examples of these instances are: a toothache, a painful bruise or sprain, a bee sting, or an ear infection during the hours when you are waiting for the antibiotic to begin to take effect.

  You should not give more than one dose of codeine unless you have consulted with a professional. Often, however, a single dose of a relatively strong pain medicine is needed to turn off a severe pain. Never give codeine to a child who has had a head injury. Never give codeine to a child with a breathing difficulty. Never give codeine to a child with a belly ache. Never give codeine to a child who may have a fracture. In all four instances, you will want to consult with a professional first to be sure that some decision is reached about the nature of the problem before the pain is dulled.

  Codeine is mildly addicting, and should be used with that in mind. It can cause dryness of the mouth, nausea, vomiting, and constipation. In large doses it can cause a depression of the breathing center of the brain, mental dullness, or sleepiness.

Codeine is given in a small dose when used to suppress a cough. As a cough remedy it usually comes in a liquid, mixed with other ingredients. Obviously, it is important not to exceed the recommended dosage. The cough-suppressant effect can also be given as plain codeine, in tablet form.

Although codeine and other opiates (such as paregoric) tend to be constipating, it is not usually a good idea to use these remedies to treat diarrhea in a child, for the drugs have too many other, undesired effects.

For pain the dosage for a child is 0.5 mgm/k, or 5 mgm/22 pounds given every four hours. The usual adult dose is 30 mgm given every four hours. Codeine is supplied in tablets containing 15 mgm; the tablets are very small but can be divided in half with fair accuracy. Therefore one can give a single dose of 7.5 mgm (half a tablet) to a child of 33 pounds, and can calculate the dose for heavier children. For smaller children one should not give codeine without consulting a professional, simply because it is very difficult to prepare the appropriate dose accurately.

For a cough the dosage is 0.167 mgm/k, or 1.67 mgm/22 pounds, given every four hours. The usual adult dose is 10 mgm given every four hours. One cannot give codeine in tablet form as a cough suppressant to a child of less than 88 pounds because it is not possible to measure such small doses with accuracy.

• Chloromycetin Ophthalmic Solution (½%). This is the antibiotic preparation commonly used to treat "pink-eye" or bacterial conjunctivitis. Bacterial conjunctivitis can be recognized as a reddening of the conjunctiva, the filmy membrane that covers the eyeball and the inside of the eyelids. The reddening is from the tiny blood vessels in the membrane becoming more visible as a result of inflammation. With a bacterial conjunctivitis there is also yellow or creamy pus that gathers in the inner corner of the eye or sometimes makes the lids stick together. Bacterial conjunctivitis is very contagious; children commonly catch it from each other at swimming pools and at schools or daycare centers.

The drops are put into the outer corner of the eye after the lids have been gently wiped clean with moistened cotton or gauze. Tears are made at the outer corner and naturally run toward the inner corner, where they drain through a tiny canal into the nose. If an eye preparation is put into the inner corner of the eye it will not bathe the whole eye. Two or three drops should be put in every 2–4 hours. It is necessary to hold the lids apart even for adults, since we have a strong blink reflex to keep things out of our eyes. If a child is struggling and protesting, mummy the child in a sheet (explained in *Skill Remedies*) or get help. Unnecessary struggling will only prolong the child's fear. Be careful not to touch the tip of the bottle to the eye, for the contents of the bottle will then be contaminated with bacteria. After treating a child for conjunctivitis, throw the rest of the remedy away on the assumption that it is probably contaminated. A similar preparation is made in ointment form, but the ointment is very difficult to put into the eyes of children and is annoying because it blurs vision.

Conjunctivitis is often an isolated infection. It can, however, be part of a more generalized infection of the respiratory system. Check for fever, cough, sinus pain, earache, and sore throat. Consult with a professional before treating conjunctivitis at home if your child seems ill with fever, earache, or a significant cough; antibiotics by mouth may be needed to help heal the infection.

- Theophylline. Theophylline is a drug related to caffeine. It has the ability to dilate the breathing tubes, and is useful therefore to treat asthma. Theophylline has other effects that are undesirable: it can cause nausea and vomiting (particularly bad for a child who has asthma, who ought not to get dehydrated) and also excitement by its action on the brain. It is essential with theophylline to give no more than the appropriate dose, and to give the remedy only when the asthma is dysfunctional or disabling. This means that a child with mild wheezing who is running around the house in vigorous play does not need theophylline; a child who is short of breath or who is sitting still and looking apprehensive about making any exertion needs treatment.

Theophylline will first be prescribed by a doctor. If you have a child with recurrent asthma you will learn, by trial and error (just as medical professionals learn about the asthma attacks of individual children), how best to treat her/him. If theophylline is part of that treatment, you can administer it at home and consult a professional only if there are new or unfamiliar symptoms or if home treatment is not making the child better.

The dosage of theophylline for a child is 3–5 mgm/K or 30–50 mgm/22 pounds, given every 6 hours. The usual adult dose is 160–400 mgm given every 6 hours. Theophylline is usually provided in a solution of 80 mgm/tablespoonful. One should begin with the lower dosage range (3 mgm/K), increasing the amount only if the lesser amount does not help, and watching always for signs of toxicity such as stomach upset and excitement. Once you have started to give the drug it should be given for one dose after the wheezing seems to be definitely resolving. Otherwise, there may appear to be a kind of rebound, the wheezing getting much worse again.

• Penicillin. Penicillin is an antibiotic, a drug that helps combat an infection caused by bacteria. Penicillin is effective against two very common bacteria that cause respiratory infections in children — the streptococcus and the pneumococcus.

Before there were antibiotics children got bacterial respiratory infections and most of them recovered with their own healing powers. It is clear that antibiotics are good to have for children who are very, very ill, as with a severe pneumonia. But it is not always clear why it is necessary for children to have penicillin for every throat or skin infection caused by the streptococcus.

A small proportion (about 3 percent) of infections by the beta-hemolytic streptococcus, if untreated, will be followed in three weeks or so by a much more serious disease, rheumatic fever. Rheumatic fever can cause permanent damage to the heart, and there is no specific curative treatment — the body must combat it as best it can. There is a smaller risk, after an untreated strep infection, of a kidney disease called glomerulonephritis, which can also leave permanent dysfunction.

Some children carry strep in their throats chronically and are not considered to be infected. Nevertheless, since penicillin is inexpensive and relatively nontoxic (except to those few persons who are allergic to the drug), it makes sense to use it to treat any ill child with a throat culture positive for beta-hemolytic strep — which is one of several varieties of strep. Most bacterial pneumonias in children past infancy, most ear infections in children past the age of 6, and most conditions of multiple skin abscesses in children also respond to penicillin.

Obviously, this is a very useful remedy for children. The most common severe side effect is allergy, usually seen first as a skin rash. If there is a strong family history of allergy or of specific allergy to penicillin, or if the child is strongly allergic to many substances, one should assume that a skin rash appearing one to ten days after beginning a course of penicillin is an indication of penicillin allergy. (A rare few persons will have a severe and immediate allergic reaction the first time they use penicillin — swelling of the breathing tubes so they have difficulty breathing, shock or a sudden drop in blood pressure so they collapse, and a severe skin reaction of hives, swelling, or peeling. More usually this severe reaction does not occur until the second or later administration of penicillin.) On the other hand, skin rashes are a common symptom in children's diseases. The fact that a skin rash occurs during a time when a child is receiving penicillin does not necessarily mean that the child is allergic to penicillin. If the rash is mild it will not be distinctive. It is also true that previously nonallergic persons can become sensitized to penicillin after taking the drug many times — still another reason not to give the drug except when it is known to be needed. If a child who is not strongly allergic to many substances and does not come from a strongly allergic family has a mild skin rash during a course of penicillin, I recommend that the drug be stopped, that another (usually less effective and more expensive) drug be substituted if the child needs it, and that penicillin be given again — only by mouth, and watching closely for the rash — on the next occasion when it appears that penicillin is the best remedy. One should never give penicillin by injection to someone who might be allergic to it, except in life-threatening situations.

Allergy to penicillin usually means allergy to several other antibiotics that are related to penicillin, such as ampicillin, cloxacillin, methicillin, and oxycillin. These are very useful and effective remedies, and we do not want to deny them to an ill person except with good reason. On the other hand, an allergic reaction can be severe, even life-threatening. Conclusion: do not give antibiotics or any other drugs unless there is good reason to do so.

A known throat or skin infection with beta-hemolytic strep is a good reason to give penicillin, because of the risk of aftereffects. When a child is ill, has had a positive throat culture for beta-hemolytic strep, and is not known to be allergic to penicillin, this remedy can wisely be given by her/his mother.

The most common side effect of penicillin is an alteration of the bacterial population in the gastrointestinal tract. We all have and need a complex and delicately balanced mixture of microorganisms residing in the gastrointestinal tract, from the mouth to the rectum. They assist in our digestion. Giving any antibiotic by mouth will change the population of microorganisms, some being killed by the drug and others, opportunistically, proliferating in greater numbers. One common pattern is that we lose a bacteria called lactobacillis and overgrow a fungus called monilia. As a consequence the mouth and tongue become sore and tender, there is diarrhea, and often a skin rash develops around the anus. Females may get an itchy vulvovaginal discharge. The easiest way to combat these troubles is to eat large quantities of yogurt, which contains lactobacillis. For those who cannot eat yogurt or for whom yogurt is not enough to offset this side effect, there are tablets or granules (called Lactinex) that will help to keep the population of lactobacillis high enough so that a monilial infection does not occur. There are also a variety of antimonilial preparations (drops for the mouth and gut, creams and ointments for the skin, and vaginal suppositories) to treat the symptoms of monilial overgrowth.

The dosage of penicillin for a child is 5–20 mgm/K, or 50–200 mgm/22 pounds given every 8 hours. The usual adult dose is 250–500 mgm, given every 8 hours. When the illness seems severe an additional dose should be given 4 hours after the first dose, to get blood levels of the drug up as quickly as possible.

Antibiotics must be given in full dosage, on schedule, and for a full course in order to rid the body of the infecting microorganism. You will thus be tied to a schedule of giving the drug every 8 hours and usually for a period of ten days. If doses are missed the bacteria can regrow and the infection may not be completely eradicated.

Penicillin is rather unstable in liquid form. It will keep for as long as ten days in the refrigerator, although it loses some of its potency toward the end. As soon as your child is old enough to swallow pills you should encourage and reward the child for taking medicine in this form. Younger children may be willing to chew pills, although they usually are somewhat bitter. Alternatively you can crush pills between two spoons and mix the powder with a little honey, jam, or granulated sugar to help the child swallow it. Pills retain their effectiveness for much longer periods of time.

Penicillin is usually supplied in tablets of 125 and 250 mgm, and in liquid preparations of 125 and 250 mgm per teaspoonful. One should not give less than the minimum dose by weight; it is safe to give a slightly higher dose, if doing so makes it easier to calculate the amount to be given.

## Over-the-Counter Drugs

Over-the-counter (OTC) drugs have been judged by the medical establishment to be safe for self-administration. There are many inconsistencies in these decisions. Sometimes low-dose tablets are available over-the-counter while high-dose tablets are available only through a prescription. This makes it possible for anyone to take enough low-dose tablets to equal a single high-dose tablet.

- Chlorpheniramine. Chlorpheniramine is one of the commonly used and somewhat effective antihistamine remedies. It is very similar to another antihistamine, brompheniramine, which is not available over-the-counter.

  The antihistamines counteract the allergic response, which is brought about in part by a substance called histamine. The antihistamines tend to dry the secretions of the respiratory tract, and also often have a sedative effect. To a lesser extent they also counteract the itch and swelling of hives, insect stings, and other skin swellings caused by allergies. For many people the most effective antihistamine for decrease of itch, respiratory drying, and sedation is diphenhydramine, also called Benadryl. The sedative effect may be desirable if you are giving the remedy to a child for itch, or to help a child sleep despite a runny nose and juicy cough. It may be much less desirable if the remedy is being given during the day. Never let a child climb trees or ride a bicycle in the street while taking an antihistamine drug until you are certain that s/he will not be unsafe as a consequence of the sedative effect of the drug. Different individuals have very different reactions to the various forms of antihistamine remedies.

Notice also that some coughs get much worse when the respiratory secretions are dried. This is especially true of coughs that are accompanied by wheezing or asthma. Never give an antihistamine remedy to anyone with a difficult asthma.

There are a variety of antihistamine preparations. Whenever this is true it means that no one preparation is entirely effective for everyone. One person will be very much helped by one remedy, while another person will be helped little if at all. Allergic symptoms, when mild and not causing significant distress, dysfunction, or disability, often call for no treatment at all — especially since treatments cost money, give side effects, and are of varying effectiveness.

The dose of chlorpheniramine for a child is 0.1 mgm/K, or 1 mgm/22 pounds, given every 6 hours. The usual dose for an adult is 4 mgm, given every 6 hours. The drug is prepared in 4 mgm tablets and also in a syrup of 2 mgm/5 cc.

• Aspirin. Aspirin remains the most effective fever- and pain-reducer. Substitutes for aspirin (the most common being acetoaminophen, which, unlike aspirin, can be prepared in liquid form) are not as effective in these two respects.

Aspirin has known side effects, and like most drugs, may be later discovered to have other side effects. A few people are allergic to aspirin. Aspirin can cause an irritation of the lining of the stomach that results in minute bleeding (or, taken chronically and in large doses, more extensive bleeding). Aspirin also affects our ability to clot blood, so that we bleed more easily from any wound. In excessive doses aspirin causes a disturbance of salt and water balance, a problem that is always more serious for children than for adults since children's bodies have a larger proportion of water than adults' bodies.

Used cautiously, only when needed, and in full and appropriate but not excessive doses, aspirin is a mainstay home remedy. It should be given on an every-four-hour schedule if needed, but one should try to give it only 4 times in 24 hours. For instance, one would not wake a sleeping child to give a dose of aspirin. If you have given 4 doses of aspirin in 24 hours for two full days and your child still needs aspirin, you should reassess the situation and think about consulting a professional about the symptom for which you are giving aspirin.

The dosage of aspirin given to a child is 10–15 mgm/K, or 100–150 mgm/22 pounds, given every 4 hours. The usual adult dose is the same. Aspirin is supplied in 75 mgm flavored tablets and in 300 mgm unflavored tablets. Either tablet may be chewed, or crushed and mixed with a sweetener. Granulated sugar, honey, jam, and applesauce are useful as sweeteners. It is not a good idea to mix any crushed tablet in a large volume of liquid (as in a four-ounce bottle of juice for a baby) because you will not be sure that all of the remedy has been taken by the child.

Aspirin has been the most common cause of poisoning in the home for children. Like all other drugs, it should be kept locked away from curious and unwary hands. The frequency of home poisonings has been significantly reduced since the introduction of safety caps for medicine bottles. BE SURE TO REPLACE THE SAFETY CAP. Children should not have access to aspirin, or any other potentially toxic remedy, without the supervision of an adult.

- Bacitracin. Bacitracin is a topical antibiotic ointment useful for treating minor skin infections. Cuts and scrapes often become mildly infected with bacteria. Our skin protects us from an invasion of infecting microorganisms, and when we break the skin we are at risk of infection. Some of us are much more susceptible to infection than others.

A slightly oozy, yellow-crusted, and very superficial skin infection is called impetigo. Because the oozing crusts are full of bacteria, the infection can easily be transmitted to other parts of the body where there are minute breaks in the skin, or to other people.

Impetigo is treated by gentle washing to remove the

crusts. This may be done with any mild soap, or with a special antibacterial soap preparation like pHisohex or Betadyne. Wash with gauze, firmly but gently, to dislodge as much of the crust as you can. Follow the washing and gentle drying with an application of Bacitracin. If your child is going to be with other children or getting dirty in play, it is a good idea to put a gauze dressing over the Bacitracin. At night, in bed, there is no reason to cover the infected place. As always, exposure to air is helpful for the healing of skin.

Most drugs applied to the skin can cause the person to develop an allergic sensitivity to that same drug if given by mouth or by injection. Bacitracin is almost never used systemically (by mouth or by injection) and is therefore safe to use on the skin. It is effective against most of the microorganisms that cause minor skin infections.

In general, it does little good to treat against an infection before the infection develops. Careful washing of skin wounds is important, as is keeping the wound clean during the interval of healing. But it is not useful to apply Bacitracin before any infection develops. You can recognize an infection by redness around the wound, increasing tenderness around the wound, and the oozing of yellow rather than clear fluid.

After 24 to 48 hours of treatment the infection should be getting better. If it is not, or if you can see a red streak running from the area of the infection toward the center of the body (called lymphangitis, an indication that the infection is being carried from the wound to the bloodstream by the lymph channels), you should consult a professional.

- Aluminum Acetate Solution (Burow's Solution). Aluminum acetate solution is a salt which is available in a dry packet, to be mixed with water. It is very helpful for treating any skin rash that is weeping, such as a rash from poison-ivy allergy.

A wet and weeping rash will clear best with the help of wet packs or soaks. Wring out clean cloths in Burow's

Solution. Put a rubber or plastic sheet under the wet packs
but do not cover them with any material that will keep the
wetness from evaporating. After a few hours of this treatment the rash should dry and begin to heal. With a small
child the treatment may last a couple of days since you
can only use the wet packs in an off-and-on fashion.

## Herbal Remedies

Some Western pharmacologists respect remedies that have
been used in many different cultures and throughout history
for their assumed assistance in healing. There is a small interest in herbal research done in other countries, and a small
interest in similar research projects in this country. But for the
most part our medical experts have ignored herbal remedies,
as they have ignored the minor but frequent and plaguing
kinds of dis-ease for which herbal remedies are most likely to
be helpful. In the meantime, we who are mothers have to cope
with the common, small, but hurtful ailments of our children.
We would do well to consider the ingenuity and caring of our
foremothers in looking for remedies that are not harmful, are
soothing, reassure our children that we care for them and know
how to make them more comfortable, and seem to do some
good.

Herbal remedies are sometimes as effective as more expensive manufactured remedies, with fewer side effects. But herbal
remedies can also be costly, and every remedy has potential
side effects. It would be especially foolish for mothers to substitute expensive and complicated regimens of herbal substances for an equally expensive and elaborate regimen of manufactured substances.

Here are some examples of herbal or natural remedies that
I have used for my own children and have recommended to
patients:

- Banana. The inside of a freshly peeled banana skin, applied to a bruise and covered with cloths wrung out in
  cool water, is said to ease the discomfort and prevent
  excessive discoloration. It can be used for a bruise any-

where on the body, including an incipient black eye, although most children very much dislike having anything put over their eyes. Don't forget to give an aspirin, if the degree of distress seems to warrant some pain remedy, and to offer the banana to eat while the dressing is having its effect!

- Peppermint. Peppermint tea is said to have properties of general physical and mental relaxation, and to work as a carminitive — acting to rid the stomach and intestine of gas. It is soothing for most belly aches.

  I first learned of this remedy not from rural or ethnic women familiar with herbal remedies but from city women who told me that the best remedy for a baby's colic was a Necco wafer (a flat white peppermint wafer manufactured by a New England candy firm); the wafer is dissolved in a four-ounce bottle of warm water. The most common kind of colic occurs in infants under 4 months, who sense the excitement and tension of older members of the household and become so wound up that they fuss and cry until they have swallowed enough air to give themselves a tense belly ache. In this situation, a peppermint drink is the most effective remedy I know of. I generally prefer a weak peppermint tea mixed with a little honey.

  A few children (often they were colicky as babies) get a tense belly ache whenever they feel stressed or upset; all of us have this symptom at one time or another. Peppermint tea (some drink it with honey, some prefer it plain) is soothing, relaxing, and seems to have a direct effect on easing a belly ache. It is best to look on the tea as an instantly helpful remedy that gives you and the child time to sit together and figure out what it was that was so upsetting and how to overcome that source of stress.

  Because aspirin so often gives a mild belly ache, peppermint tea is much more helpful for stress-related symptoms like headache and stomach ache than is aspirin.

- Cabbage leaves. The flat, soft leaf of a cabbage, bound onto an insect bite with a cool damp cloth, seems to relieve the sting and reduce the inflammation. Again we have a condition that is mild but annoying, enough to cause a child tears and warranted self-pity, a situation that we ought to respond to with help or a suggestion for self-treatment. This is a remedy that children can and do apply for themselves.

- Aloe. The aloe plant grows easily as a houseplant. A broken leaf oozes a clear, gelatinlike substance that is very soothing for skin irritations like minor burns and scrapes. Be sure to wash the wound well, with plenty of running water (more important than the kind of soap used), before rubbing on the aloe. If the hurt is still painful, covering it with a nonstick dressing (called Telfa) will keep the air away and take away most of the sting.

- Cayenne. Cayenne pepper, like other hot spices, causes one to perspire. Perspiration is one of the mechanisms by which the body copes with fever, for air-cooling on wet skin helps the body bring down its internal temperature. This diaphoretic effect (causing perspiration) is shared by thyme, nutmeg, and ginger, among other herbs and spices. A tea made of some mixture of these ingredients and sweetened with honey is very soothing for a child with a fever.

## Skill Remedies

Much of the work done by doctors and nurses to assist in the minor and common dis-eases of children is simple and can be done at home. Most of these skills are not put down on paper; they are taught by demonstration and explanation as part of medical training. They could easily be learned by mothers and done at home.

In the section that follows I try to explain in words what is better shown in demonstration. These, again, are examples only. Ask to have procedures explained to you when you bring a child to an emergency room or a clinic. Unless elaborate or special equipment is needed, you can probably do the procedure yourself at home.

*How to "mummy" a child.* If you must do something to a child who is frightened or protesting, you will begin by trying

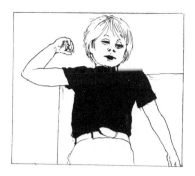

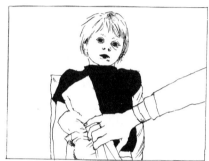

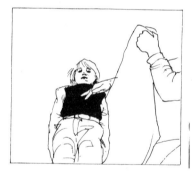

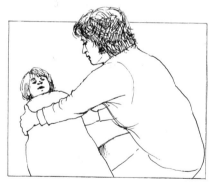

### "MUMMYING" A CHILD

1) Lay the child with right arm at right edge of the sheet
2) Sheet is drawn over the left arm, under body, and up between body and right arm
3) Sheet goes around right arm and back under the body
4) The rest of the sheet is wrapped around the child's body at bottom

to soothe and explain. Young children who don't use language well will not be very comforted by explanations. Generally, the longer the child anticipates in fear, the more panicky s/he will be. In this situation it is kindest to use swift and effective restraint, and get done what you have to get done. (An example: examining a child's eye to be sure that it has not been injured by a scratch or a blow.)

To mummy a child, fold a sheet lengthwise into a strip a little less wide than the child is tall. Lay one end of the strip on a bed or table, lying horizontally. Lay the child on the end of the strip so that her/his shoulders are even with the top edge of the strip and the vertical edge is under the left arm. Pull the long end of the strip up between the right arm and body, then wrap the strip over the right arm and under the back. Bring the strip up between the left arm and body, then over the left arm and under the back. The remaining end of the strip is wrapped around and around the child's body.

With a light child of 35 pounds or less this maneuver can be done quickly by one person. Practice it when you don't need it, when it can be a game for you and the child. With a heavier child who is struggling you may need help with the wrapping. It is very secure and not unpleasant for the child, except for the indignity of being restrained. In general, the indignity of restraints at a hospital or clinic is so much more demeaning to the child that it is a kindness to do whatever needs to be done at home.

*How to examine an eye for a scratch.* An eye poked with a stick or other scratchy object is a common accident for children. If the child's complaints stop immediately and you are not sure that the object actually touched the eye, you probably need not worry. But if the child continues to complain, or holds the eye shut, or if the eye is tearing, there may have been some damage to the cornea, the covering of the pupil and lens. Fluoresceine is a dye that is sold in small paper-impregnated strips. This dye has the specific property of staining damaged places on the surface of the cornea a brilliant, fluorescent green.

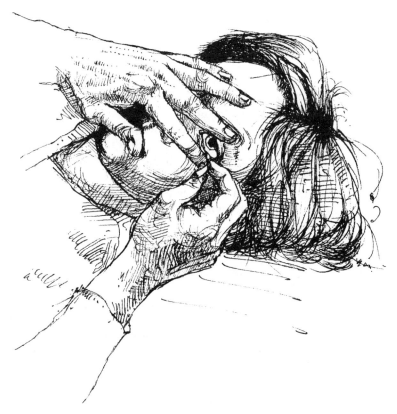

Using a fluoresceine dye strip to examine the eye for a corneal abrasion

Touch one end of a paper strip to the pool of tears in the lower outer corner of the eye. The tears will stain with the dye and will wash across the eye. After a moment, examine the surface of the eyeball with the lights in the room turned down low and holding a bright flashlight to the side of the eye. You may see tiny bright green dots, or even long green tracks. These are scratches on the surface of the cornea. A brightly stained ring with a dot in the center may mean that a foreign body is embedded in the cornea.

If the scratch marks are small and the child's complaints

are minimal, cover the eye with a sterile eye pad secured with Scotch tape to the forehead and cheek for a period of 6 to 10 hours. When you remove the pad the symptoms of pain and tearing should be gone.

If there appears to be a foreign body, if the scratch marks are large, if the pain is severe, or if vision seems to be diminished or blurred, have the child checked by a professional. Similarly, if covering the eye does not ease the pain and the child continues to complain, take the child to a professional. Although an eye doctor may do nothing more than put on a patch and let the child's eye heal itself, this is an instance when you will want the professional to take part of the responsibility for the outcome.

*How to close a laceration.* A laceration is a cut through the skin. The two edges of the skin pull apart, and between them you can see granules of fat. If the two edges of the skin do not pull apart the wound is a scratch and needs only to be cleaned and covered to protect it from dirt.

If the laceration is very long, if the two edges cannot be pulled together easily, or if you can see muscle at the bottom of the laceration, it should be stitched together. If the laceration is in the hand, always check with a professional. A tendon (the fibrous end of a muscle) might have been cut, resulting in an inability to make certain hand movements. If the laceration is on the face you might want to have very fine sewing (plastic surgery) to minimize the scar that always forms in healing.

Many of the lacerations that children get are small and can be taped together at home. You should have on hand some antiseptic soap (like pHisohex or Betadyne), tincture of benzoin, and butterfly bandaids. Wash the laceration well with a solution of the soap. Examine the laceration closely after it has been washed and dried. If it has dirt or pieces of glass imbedded in it, have a professional anesthetize it and remove the foreign particles. If it appears clean and is not in an area where a small scar will be of great importance, you can take care of it and avoid the needle pricks of local anesthesia and of suturing. (In the kind of laceration described above, the doctor in an emergency room will probably do exactly as you are going to do at home.)

Dry the edges of the laceration very carefully. With a cotton-tipped swab, paint the edges of the laceration with the benzoin; wait five minutes and paint again. The partially dried

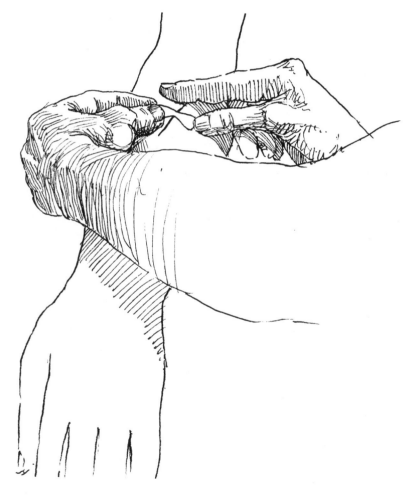

Taping a laceration with a butterfly bandaid

benzoin is a sticky film to which the tape ends of the bandaids
will stick firmly. Pull the middle of the two edges of the laceration together, overlapping a little, and secure them with a
butterfly. Put on as many butterflies as needed to hold the
whole length of the laceration together. Because the butterflies
are narrow in the center, the laceration itself will not be entirely covered with tape.

Check your child's immunization record. If the child is
less than 5 and has not had a tetanus injection within the last
two months, s/he should have one now. If the child is older
than 5 and has had a tetanus booster within the last ten years
s/he does not need another booster now. If the laceration is
extensive and s/he has not had a booster in more than five
years s/he may need another booster. In that case, however,
you will already be consulting with a professional.

The butterfly dressing should stay on for about a week.
Keep the taped laceration clean and dry. Uncover it at night
when the child is sleeping so that it is exposed to the air.
Check it daily for signs of infection: a surrounding area of
redness, increasing tenderness, and/or an oozing of pus. If the
butterflies come off before the week is over and the edges of
the laceration do not look securely regrown together, the butterflies can be reapplied.

Scar formation is mostly a matter of individual chemistry.
Some of us make large scars with the finest plastic surgery,
while others make very small scars. With children, a scar will
continue to get smaller and less visible for a period of two
years or so. For simple lacerations, there will be no more scar
with a butterfly closure than with suturing.

Don't forget to give the child aspirin if the laceration is
painful. And don't forget to offer her/him an especially nutritious diet to assist in healing.

*How to dress a burn.* A first-degree burn is red and may
be slightly raised, like a sunburn. A second-degree burn blisters; the blister may stay intact or may break so that the top
layer of skin falls in shreds. A third-degree burn destroys the
entire skin in all its layers, is markedly swollen, and appears

white or black. Unlike first- and second-degree burns, a third-degree burn is usually not painful except at its edges.

All third-degree burns, and all first- and second-degree burns that cover more than 10 percent of the body, should be evaluated and treated by a professional. In an adult, for reference, a burn over an entire arm would be 7 percent of body surface area; an entire upper leg varies in its proportion of surface area from 6 percent of a newborn to 9 percent of a 10-year-old. First- and second-degree burns that cover small areas can be treated at home.

The pain of a burn, after the initial insult, comes mostly from exposure to air. Wash the burn under cold running water until the first pain stops. Get help if the child cannot hold the burn under the running water, for you will want to cover the burn as soon as it is taken out of the water. Get together sterile gauze impregnated with petroleum jelly or Betadyne and some springy gauze outer wrapping called Kerlex. Quickly pat dry the skin around the burn. Cover the burn with the Vasoline or Betadyne gauze, handling the gauze as little as possible to avoid contamination with bacteria. Cover the area with Kerlex, wound many times around the burn, which acts as a bumper dressing.

The pain should diminish within an hour. Change the dressing every day. When the child says that the burned area no longer hurts, you need not replace the dressing. Be very respectful of blisters — they are a kind of natural bandage, protecting the new skin underneath that needs time to toughen up before it is exposed to bacteria.

These examples of substance and skill remedies should give you ideas about how to apply specific remedies in specific situations. As your children grow, you will continue to learn new and different home-remedy procedures.

Here is a list of supplies that you might keep handy. It would be sensible if more than one household shared this store of equipment and supplies. A community center might serve as a central location, from which these items could be obtained for use.

1. Ace bandage
2. A mild steroid ointment (by prescription)
3. Aspirin or aspirin substitute
4. Bacitracin ointment
5. Betadyne or pHisohex soap (by prescription)
6. Bloodpressure apparatus — cuffs of 7, 12, and 18 centimeter width
7. Burow's Solution
8. Butterfly bandaids
9. Camomile tea
10. Centrifuge (for hematocrit)
11. Chlorpheniramine (if your family has bothersome allergies)
12. Codeine — 2 tabs (by prescription)
13. Fluoresceine strips
14. Ipecac Syrup (by prescription)
15. Ipsatol Cough Remedy
16. Kerlex bandage
17. Labstix
18. Lancet, swabs, glass tubes (for hematocrit)
19. Nonallergenic tape
20. Otoscope
21. Peppermint tea
22. Rectal thermometer
23. Regular Band-Aids
24. Rosehip tea, containing vitamin C
25. Scotch tape
26. Stethoscope
27. Sterile gauze pads — small and large
28. Stresstabs — high potency Vitamin B tablets
29. Telfa pads
30. Throat culture materials
31. Tincture of Benzoin
32. Uricult Kits
33. Vasoline
34. Vitamin C tablets (if this seems to help members of your family recover from upper respiratory infections)
35. Vitamin E capsules

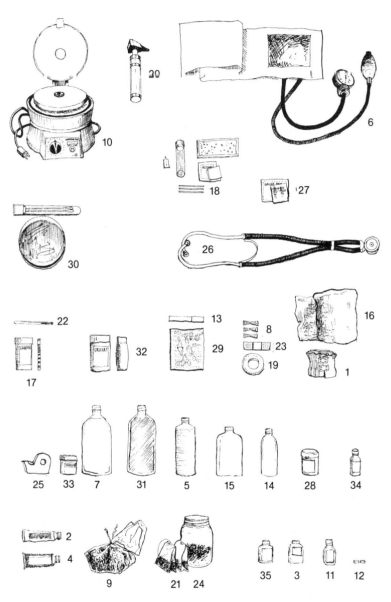

A community kit of medical supplies (see text for identification of items)

# CHAPTER 5

# Common Illnesses and Injuries

This chapter gives information about some of the kinds of dis-ease that are common in childhood. In each instance, the kind of information discussed is helpful for mothers to know, both in the interests of helping the child heal his/her body and also in the giving of informed and appropriate care. For each instance of dis-ease you will want to know:

- Personal symptoms — how the problem came about. This you can learn by finding out what complaints the child has, and how s/he feels (the subjective information or history). If the child is an infant, you must depend on your own interpretation of symptoms.
- Physical signs — what the problem looks like. This you can determine by examining the child — looking, feeling, listening, smelling, tasting (the objective information or physical exam).
- Other information that you might need to consider before deciding how to proceed.
- Remedies to be applied.

This is certainly not a complete listing, nor is it meant to be. The illnesses and injuries that have been chosen for discussion are examples of the dis-ease that children frequently have, of the sort that mothers commonly care for at home. The discussions are examples of the kinds of information that mothers need in order to give responsible and competent care.

The purpose of the chapter is not to teach everything that you need to know, but to suggest a way for you to think about and to understand your child when s/he is sick. Information of this sort should be available to you about any illness or injury that your child might have. You can get this sort of information from nurses, doctors, and other medical professionals, from medical textbooks, and from other mothers who have taken care of children with dis-ease similar to what your child is experiencing.

**Anemias**

Hemoglobin is the substance of the body that carries oxygen to every tissue; it is contained in the red cells of the blood. When a child is deficient in hemoglobin s/he is said to be anemic.

*Personal symptoms.* An anemic child may be fatigued chronically and inexplicably. A relative lack of oxygen can slow all body processes. Children who are anemic may also be susceptible to infection. Some anemic children become finicky eaters, turning away from the very foods that they need to rebuild their stores of hemoglobin.

*Physical signs.* Anemic children look pale. Their pallor can be seen on the skin and also on the mucous membranes, for instance in the mouth. If the reason for the anemia is that red cells are breaking down at a faster rate than usual, one may be able to feel the liver and/or spleen (organs that break red cells and process the products of that breakdown) on examining the belly. Other physical signs accompanying anemia are related to the reason for the anemia. There may be enlarged lymph nodes, a jaundiced or yellow color to the skin (from blood breakdown), joint swellings, or a variety of other signs. In severe anemia the heart rate may be increased. Anemias are determined by measuring the hemoglobin in the blood, or by estimating the number and volume of red cells in a test called the hematocrit (see Chapter 3, section on Blood Tests). Other laboratory tests may be needed to determine the reason for the anemia.

*Other things you should know.* There are a variety of causes of anemia. Some are the inherited peculiarities of an individual's hemoglobin; some are the result of poisonings, as with lead; some are the result of inflammatory or infectious disease; some result from a lack of a particular nutrient needed by the body to manufacture hemoglobin.

By far the most common reason for anemia in children is iron deficiency. Children have relatively few reserves of iron (and most other substances) because they are small. They may not take in enough iron in their food for a variety of reasons — because iron-rich foods are not being offered, because of food-finickyness or disputes with a parent about who is going to decide what they eat, or because they are filling up on other foods that are not rich in iron (like cookies and milk) so that their small appetites have no room left for foods that are more nutritious. Some children do not seem to absorb iron as well as others and need to eat extra amounts of iron-rich foods. Children with iron-deficiency anemia often develop a transiently dysfunctional iron absorption, so that even the iron they do take in is not absorbed efficiently into the bloodstream.

Adults have higher hemoglobin levels and hematocrits than children do. Doctors differ in the interpretation of a "low"-level hemoglobin for a child (the level at which a child should be treated). There is a good reason not to give a child excessive amounts of iron. Some superfluous iron can be stored in the liver. There is a condition, now seen most commonly in adults, of iron overload. This is when the liver can no longer work properly because it is sodden with stored iron. One can always offer a child more of the foods that are rich in iron and trust that a child will not eat iron in excess. It would be difficult to overload a child with iron by feeding him/her too many iron-rich foods. But one should not give extra additive or medicinal iron to children unless there is a good reason for doing so. A good reason would be a valid and reliable test indicating low hemoglobin, or a marginal test with some signs and symptoms (pallor, fatigue, a series of contagious infections) that suggest that the child is not doing well because of a mild anemia.

*Remedies.* Iron-deficiency anemia is so common that, in the absence of any signs or symptoms that suggest another cause for the anemia, the first remedy is a so-called therapeutic trial of iron. One would have a professional investigate the cause of an anemia, before giving iron, if the child showed symptoms of acute illness — sudden sleepiness or fatigue, irritability, fever, or complaints of pain; enlarged lymph nodes; signs of easy bleeding; or, in extreme anemia, a very rapid heart rate, extreme pallor or fatigue.

If none of these signs or symptoms is evident, begin the remedy by reviewing the child's diet. Foods rich in iron are red meats, eggs, dried fruits, legumes and whole grains, and dark green leafy vegetables. Is the child eating foods, other than these, in excess — too much refined sugar or large quantities of milk? (A child between the ages of 18 months and 5 years with a finicky appetite should not drink more than a pint of milk a day.)

If the hematocrit is only one or two percentage points less than expected (see Chapter 4, ●Hematocrit) one may be able to correct the anemia by improving the child's diet. If food choice is a battleground for the child, or if the anemia is more severe, the child should take medicinal iron. Fer-in-Sol is a liquid iron preparation, given in a dose of 15 mgm of elemental iron (0.6 cc) four times a day between meals. Older children who can swallow capsules can take iron sulfate in capsule form (60 mgm of elemental iron per capsule) two or three times a day between meals. The dose is 6 mgm/k, or 60 mgm/22 pounds, given every day.

Whether you begin to treat the anemia by diet or by diet and medicinal iron, the hemoglobin or hematocrit level should be checked again in three weeks to be sure that the anemia is improving with this treatment. By either measurement, the hemoglobin should be at normal levels by this time. Treatment with medicinal iron should continue for two full months, to replenish iron stores. Treatment with diet should, of course, be lifelong. If your child has been a poor eater, you can expect that his/her appetite for nutritious foods will increase at about the time that the hemoglobin level returns to normal.

If the hemoglobin does not return to normal after three weeks of treatment with medicinal iron, you should consult a professional. If the anemia is not corrected after three weeks of an improved diet, you should treat with medicinal iron and check the hemoglobin level again in another three weeks — assuming, of course, that the child still seems well.

## Appendicitis

The appendix is a little finger of bowel tissue that protrudes from the main body of the bowel at the point where the many feet of small bowel join the beginning of the colon, or large bowel. The appendix has no function for us, although it served a purpose in the animals from which we are descended. Because it is a blind pouch, it can become clogged, inflamed, infected, and swollen. If this happens it can cause a blockage of the bowel at the point where it is joined. This condition of inflammation of the appendix is called appendicitis.

*Personal symptoms.* A child with appendicitis will appear listless and will complain of a belly ache. These indicators of appendicitis, like all of those listed below, are somewhat irregular and unreliable. The only certain way of diagnosing appendicitis is by a surgical procedure, opening the belly and removing the appendix so that it can be examined under a microscope. The symptoms listed here are all typical of appendicitis, but no one symptom is necessary in order to think that appendicitis is the most likely explanation of the child's distess.

The belly ache of appendicitis is, in many cases, first indicated by the child as being around the belly button. This is probably because children are not very good at localizing pain in the belly area (or anywhere else) and the belly button is a handy landmark to focus on. The pain may come and go but gradually it increases in intensity and in specific localization, so that finally the child indicates that the hurt is in the right lower part of the abdomen.

Other symptoms of appendicitis are probably related to the degree of bowel blockage, however mild. The child is not hungry and may complain of nausea. There may be vomiting, and an expected bowel movement may not have been passed.

As time goes on, usually over a period of less than 24 hours, there will probably be a low-grade fever — a degree or so above normal. The belly ache may hurt less when the child lies curled in a ball. S/he may walk with a limp. The pain may increase in intensity, as may all other symptoms.

*Physical signs.* Examination of a child suspected of having appendicitis follows the same orderly routine of any other examination. A child who complains or appears ill should always have ears, throat, neck, nodes, lungs, skin, and belly examined. The examination of the belly, as always, should be done with the child lying on his/her back, knees bent up and hands at the side. Deep breathing with the mouth open also helps the child relax the belly muscles, partly by giving the child something else to think about. Always feel the belly first in those areas that you think are not tender, leaving to last the area that you suspect of tenderness. Otherwise, the child will tense with the tenderness and it will be more difficult to examine the rest of the abdomen.

The pain and tenderness of appendicitis should become more marked and more localized over time. This means that you will want to do several examinations to gauge change over time. The point of tenderness when the appendix is inflamed will be found approximately at the third angle of an equal-sided triangle with the other angles at the belly button and the crest of the hipbone.

When you listen to the belly with a stethoscope you may hear normal bowel sounds or, if there is some blockage of the bowel, the quiet or tinkling rushes that are characteristic of bowel obstruction.

If any symptoms of appendicitis exist and go on for as long as 12 hours, and if there are no other signs of some alternative illness that explain the child's discomfort, a medical professional should be consulted. You may want to consult professional opinion before that time if the child's distress is extreme.

*Other things you should know.* Some common illnesses

that resemble appendicitis are strep throat (which in a school-aged child, especially, can cause as much belly ache as sore throat), pneumonia, constipation, urinary-tract infections, and viral infections (including mononucleosis) that cause tender enlargement of the lymph nodes in the belly. In an adolescent girl, ovulation — approximately two weeks after her last menstrual period — can result in a tiny bit of bleeding that causes pain in the lower part of the belly.

Pneumonia can be identified by a chest X-ray. A strep throat can be identified (after waiting 24 hours) by a throat culture. A urine infection can be identified by a microscopic urinalysis (looking at the urine for white blood cells, a sign of infection, and for bacteria) and by a urine culture, which can be read after 18 hours. Mononucleosis can be identified by specific laboratory tests (see section on Mononucleosis) but these tests are not often positive at the beginning of the illness. Other viral illnesses that cause a tender enlargement of the abdominal lymph nodes are less easy to identify with certainty, although usually the white blood count is different for a viral illness than it is for appendicitis. Constipation can sometimes be identified by experienced examination of the belly, but it should not cause a rise in temperature or the changes in the white blood count seen in the examination of the blood.

The laboratory indicators of appendicitis are an elevated white blood count in the blood, and a relative increase and immaturity of the polymorphonuclear white cells, the cells that the body calls forth to deal with bacterial infection. At the same time there should be no strong indication from examination of the urine that there is a urine infection, and no indication on chest X-ray that there is a pneumonia.

The absolute diagnostic test for appendicitis is the examination under the microscope of the tissue of the appendix. If appendicitis goes on unrecognized for some time, there is a chance that the appendix will burst or rupture and the infection within the space of the appendix will be spilled into the abdominal cavity. In this case, there will be a generalized infection in the belly, an inflamation of the membrane that lines the belly cavity, called peritonitis. This is a serious and sometimes life-threatening infection. For this reason, and because the appendix is an organ that has no function for human beings, surgeons are rather eager to operate whenever they think that appendicitis might exist.

*Remedies.* The remedy for appendicitis is to make a small incision in the belly, find and cut off the appendix, sew up the small hole in the bowel that has been created, and close up the hole in the skin. This is a relatively easy operation for a healthy child to endure. It is a much easier experience than waiting until the inflamed appendix has ruptured, combating the infection in the belly cavity, and then operating to remove the infected and burst appendix.

On the other hand, there is always some risk associated with general anesthesia. No one should be submitted to major surgery with anesthesia unless there is some rational and explainable reason for the procedure. The risk of death from general anesthesia is less than one-tenth of one percent. Most anesthesia deaths occur in the old or the debilitated, at small rural hospitals that do not have recently trained anesthesiologists, and in patients who are having lengthy and physiologically challenging surgery. Nonetheless, major surgery is never a totally benign experience.

A child who is suspected of having appendicitis should be followed by a professional for several hours before a decision to recommend surgery is made. In a few rare cases, a surgeon will believe that rupture of the appendix is imminent and will recommend immediate surgery on the strength of first findings in the physical examination and the laboratory studies. In the more usual case, the surgeon will want the child to eat or drink nothing by mouth (in case a general anesthesia is going to be administered) for a period of a few hours, while repeated physical examinations are done and laboratory studies are performed. This waiting-and-watching period is often passed with the child's being admitted to the hospital as an inpatient. Alternatively, if you are willing to deny food and drink to the child and to take the child repeatedly to the emergency room, s/he can remain at home during the period of observation.

An appendectomy performed on a healthy child, in a hospital with a competent anesthesiologist, by a surgeon you trust, with your participation as mother maximized by hospital policy, can be a positive and growth-promoting experience for child and mother alike. The experiences surrounding the removal of the appendix can be taken as opportunities for learning, comfort, and closeness. The child's recovery is likely to be prompt, easy, and healthful.

## Asthma

Asthma is a constriction of the breathing tubes that results in difficulty in breathing out, called wheezing.

*Personal symptoms.* Asthma seems to be increasing as a dysfunctional complaint of children who live in cities, probably as a result of the damage done to the respiratory system by constant exposure to chemically polluted air.

Some children have only one or two episodes of asthma, usually as part of a specific and limited bacterial or viral respiratory infection. Other children wheeze frequently, with infection and without; many of these latter children have family histories of allergic tendencies, and some have other evidence in their own lives of allergic responses, such as eczema or hives or hay fever. For children who tend to wheeze, even changes in temperature or humidity, unaccustomed exertion, and emotion-laden experiences can bring on an attack of asthma.

For each child who wheezes frequently, there develops a pattern of onset, response to treatment, and self-healing. The pattern changes slowly over time — the wheezing of infants is usually not in the same form as the wheezing in adolescents — but the pattern remains typical for the individual child. For some, there is a warning symptom or sign — irritability, cough, or a fall in appetite. Wheezing episodes can be preceded by fever, the wheezing can begin as fever begins, or fever may be a later happening. Many children who wheeze have little or no fever, even with bacterial infections which, in most children, would cause at least a moderate rise in body temperature.

There is usually a frequent, nonproductive cough when wheezing is well established.

The presence of bacterial infection as a precipitating factor in wheezing episodes can be discovered by reviewing the child's known exposure to contagious disease, especially illness in other family members that seems to be of bacterial origin by its course and because it appears to respond to antibiotic treatment. The giving of antibiotics to an asthmatic child, noting the apparent response of the illness, is helpful in determining whether bacterial infection is a regular precipitant for that child. Response to antibiotics usually occurs not immediately but after 12 to 48 hours of taking the drug, and is characteristically a sharp and dramatic recovery or diminution of symptoms and signs of the illness.

For some children, significant and disabling attacks of asthma are triggered by environmental changes (cold or dryness), exposure to dust or allergenic foods, or emotionally upsetting events. Often more than one precipitant is involved in the characteristic pattern.

Some children with asthma clear their wheezing readily with a few treatments, showing marked improvement after the initial doses of medications. Others need a combination of emotional support, comforting remedies, and multiple doses of medicines directed to the constriction of the breathing tubes, and show only slow improvement over many hours or even days. Individual children require different patterns of convalescence, as well.

In second and later episodes of wheezing, you will become very knowledgeable about your child's pattern of illness. At each episode, you will want to review what you know about the possibility of an inhaled foreign body lodged in the breathing tubes; the possibility of exposure to a bacterial or viral respiratory infection; the possibility of exposure to some specific triggering substance to which the child has a marked allergy, such as cat fur; and the possibility of an emotionally distressing event in the child's life.

*Physical signs.* While wheezing can usually be recognized by simply looking and listening to the child, initially you will want to listen carefully with a stethoscope to determine the differences between asthmatic breathing and the child's normal breathing. In asthma the expiratory phase of breathing is prolonged and strained. There are sounds during expiration, typically a whistling or sighing, that reflect the effort to push air out. With severe asthma there may be a grunt at the end of expiration. When you listen with the stethoscope there may be inspiratory wheezing as well, but the prolongation of the expiratory phase of breathing is unmistakable.

Observe the child carefully. If s/he is running around and playing as usual, the wheezing is not compromising his/her breathing to any significant extent. This does not mean that it does not need treatment. If s/he tries to play and then has to rest for breath, s/he is experiencing significant disability.

When wheezing is severe, children will sit or lie very quietly. As wheezing increases in intensity so that the exchange of oxygen and other gases in the lungs is compromised, their color will become ashen and they may become agitated and restless. Severe wheezing will also cause the movements of the chest that accompany breathing to change. Exertion of the accessory muscles of breathing — the small muscles between the ribs and just above the clavicle or collarbone — will be evident as the respiratory effort increases. The nose may flare widely with inspiration. The rate of breathing will increase as well, as the child works harder to take in oxygen and to get rid of waste gases.

Examine the child carefully for other evidence of respiratory infection — enlarged nodes in the neck, reddened eardrums, a reddened throat. Look for other signs of allergic response on the skin — hives or eczema.

Keep a record of vital signs — heart rate, breathing rate, and temperature. Until and unless you feel confident that the wheezing episode can be easily cared for at home without complications, information about progression of the child's breathing distress should be recorded to guide later treatment.

*Remedies.* If your child's wheezing is sometimes set off by bacterial respiratory infection, you will want to consult a professional about the advisability of giving antibiotics. Giving antibiotics to your child will depend on the course of the wheezing episode and what you have observed in your examination.

The two routine home remedies that should be started at the first sign of wheezing are the increase of fluid intake, and the moistening of the air that the child breathes by running a cool mist vaporizer. Along with the constriction of the breathing tubes that makes breathing out so difficult, there is characteristically a drying of the respiratory secretions so that they interfere with or block the expiration of air from the lungs. Increasing moisture inside and outside the child's body tends to loosen these secretions. Do not ever give antihistamines to a child who is wheezing. Children who have asthma may also have difficulty with a chronic stuffy nose — often on an allergic basis. Antihistamines may be recommended to treat the stuffy nose, for their effect of drying respiratory secretions. But, it is obvious that the drying effect will make wheezing worse.

The fluids given to the child should be dictated by the child's wishes. Breathing difficulties can cause changes in the composition of gases dissolved in the blood. This can, in turn, alter the balance of salts in the blood. If the child firmly indicates that s/he would like something particular to drink, s/he may well need the salt-balance characteristic of that fluid.

There are two simple first-line drug remedies for the constriction of the breathing tubes. One is a drug that you will keep at home for a child who has recurrent difficulties with wheezing, called theophylline. Theophylline needs to be given in full doses (see section on Theophylline) but not in excess of the full dose, for it is a drug with a narrow margin between helpful and toxic effects. In excessive doses it can cause agitation, irritability, and also vomiting, all of which are specifically troubling for a wheezing child who needs to be calm and comforted and needs to retain body fluids. For most children, theophylline is given every 6 hours for 48 hours, lest there be an apparent rebound effect when the drug is stopped early in the course of the asthmatic episode.

The other remedy is given by injection, which means a trip to a medical facility unless you learn to give the injection at home. The drug is called epinephrine, and it has an almost immediate effect of dilating the breathing tubes. Because it is given by injection, and because it often has side effects of tremor, a rapid heartbeat, sweating, and anxiety, it is useful only to alter the pattern of wheezing for a child who is in acute distress. Its effects wear off in a few hours, so that it is most useful as a dramatic, one-time reliever of the wheezing, which can have a significant, psychologically comforting effect on the child. Unless wheezing is really disabling, epinephrine should not be given. It can be given in long-acting form (the drug is called Sus-phrine) for children who need it and who do not have unpleasant side effects from it. If your child regularly needs epinephrine in either of its forms, you should consider learning the simple technique of giving the subcutaneous injections.

Long-range treatment of asthma might include, for an individual child, allergic testing and desensitization, attention to sources of emotional stress, and avoidance of known precipitants such as dust, dry air, cold, or exposure to air. It has been demonstrated that a regular program of exercise, graded so that the child develops an increasing respiratory competence in extreme exertion, is very helpful for children who have chronic or recurrent asthma.

Although a small number of children die in severe asthmatic attacks, most asthmatic children do well, rarely need more than home-based treatment, and eventually "grow out of" their asthmatic tendencies. Only about 10 percent of asthmatic children will continue with severe symptoms when they are adults. More than half will have no difficulty with asthma by the time they are grown.

### Chicken Pox

. Chicken pox (varicella) is a highly contagious viral illness characterized by fever and a distinctive rash.

*Personal symptoms.* The incubation period for chicken pox is one and one-half to three weeks. You may know about a specific exposure to chicken pox, or you may have heard that there have been cases of chicken pox at your child's school. On the other hand, since the illness is so remarkably contagious, the exposure may have been quite incidental (in the grocery store or on a bus, for instance), and the appearance of the disease may come as a surprise to all. The virus of chicken pox is the same as the virus that causes shingles in older persons, so that a child can come down with chicken pox after exposure to an adult with shingles, and a grandparent or other adult could develop shingles after exposure to your child with chicken pox. As with most viral illnesses, the time of maximum contagiousness is at the end of the incubation period, just before symptoms of the illness begin to appear.

The interval between the first appearance of symptoms and the appearance of the rash is brief, only a few hours. This is always a difficult time for everyone who helps with healing; it is apparent that the child is ill, probable that before long some more clear-cut symptoms and signs will appear, but quite unknown for the time exactly what the illness will be. All one can do is wait and watch carefully, not giving any remedies that might cloud evidence of the illness. Children begin their experience with chicken pox, usually, with fever, droopiness, some loss of appetite, and crankiness.

Soon the rash begins to appear. It usually starts on the trunk and spreads to the head and down the arms and legs. The pox affect not only all of the skin, including the scalp — the hands and feet are least affected — but also the mucous membranes of the mouth and the entire gastrointestinal tract, including the anus. In girls the mucous membranes of the vulva may also be affected.

The pox are intensely itchy, especially in children older than 10. Before this age the nerves that carry the signals of pain (itch is a mild form of pain) are not fully mature, and the degree of itchiness is variable. In infants, itch may appear to be no problem at all. The pox in the mucous membranes of the mouth and the gastrointestinal tract cause pain, shown by complaints of a sore mouth and refusal to drink, and complaints of belly ache. There may be vomiting or diarrhea. The younger the child, the more likely that gastrointestinal complaints and discomforts will be a problem.

The fever remains as long as new pox are breaking out. There are three rather rare complications of chicken pox, and any of the three may be signaled by the *return* of fever. One is the development of a significant amount of bacterial infection in the pox, as a result of scratching. The second complication is viral pneumonia, signaled by a cough and some difficulty breathing. The third is meningoencephalitis, signaled by irritability or sleepiness and a headache. It is probable, however, that many children with chicken pox have some mild degree of meningoencephalitis. But it is difficult to make a certain diagnosis of this condition since complaints of headaches are frequent; sleepiness may be a reaction to fever, and irritability may be a response to the itch and pain caused by the pox.

*Physical signs.* The rash of chicken pox has an absolutely typical appearance. Lesions appear in crops in all affected areas; new lesions continue to appear for a few hours, at least, and often for several days. Each pox begins as a flat red spot. It soon becomes raised, and then develops into a small blister filled with clear fluid. The blister then develops a milky appearance and soon ruptures, drying into a scab. What is also typical of chicken pox is that after the first few hours of the illness one can see, in any involved area of the body, pox in all stages of development — some flat red spots, some raised red spots, some clear blisters, some milky blisters, and some scabs.

In addition to observing the character and progression of the rash, one should watch for indications of the most frequent complications of the illness. Bacterial infection in the pox is seen when the blisters develop a yellow, pussy appearance with a surrounding ring of red inflammation; ordinarily, by the time the blisters (also called vesicles) have become milky most of the redness has gone. Infected pox are more likely to develop into scars. If many pox are infected the child may develop a bloodstream bacterial infection, a more serious complication. A few infected pox are usual, but if many are infected, or if the fever reappears after the period of development of new pox, one should consult a professional to consider specific antibiotic treatment for the bacterial infection.

Chicken-pox pneumonia can develop at any time during the illness. It is signaled by a cough. Listening with a stethoscope one can hear the usual signs of pneumonia, rales and perhaps some wheezing. Unless there is secondary lung infection with bacteria, there is no specific treatment for chicken-pox pneumonia; telephone consultation with a professional is probably sufficient to alert your medical back-up to the presence of the complication. As long as the child breathes comfortably and facial color remains good, home care is quite sufficient. Pneumonia is a more common complication of chicken pox in teenagers and adults, less common in younger children.

Meningoencephalitis also has no specific treatment, and can be cared for at home unless signs and symptoms are severe. Check to be sure that the child's neck bends forward comfortably and is not stiff. Reappearance of high fever after the rash has broken out, with complaints of severe headache or extreme irritability and/or sleepiness, forceful vomiting, and the absence of bacterial infection in the pox or pneumonia, would make one suspect a more than usual degree of meningoencephalitis.

*Other things you should know.* Persons with chronic disease and those whose immune systems are compromised (such as those who are taking steroid drugs for any reason) can become seriously ill with chicken pox or shingles. Otherwise, exposure to chicken pox may be no particular problem. Be sure to notify others who may come into contact with your child of the illness, and let them decide whether they want to be exposed. Because chicken pox is usually a more mild illness in early childhood than in the years after adolescence, and because almost all of us will experience this illness at some time, many mothers will feel all right about exposing their children.

Other children in your own household who have not yet had chicken pox will usually come down with the illness in due time. The description given above fits the usual case of chicken pox; a very few children have only one or two pox, a very mild fever, and an illness of only a day or two. If a child has had two household exposures to chicken pox and has not developed the florid disease, it seems safe to assume that that child has already had chicken pox in a mild and inapparent form.

*Remedies.* Aspirin is a standby remedy for chicken pox — it helps with the fever, with the pain of the pox in the gastrointestinal tract, and with the itch. Be sure to try to limit aspirin dosage to 4 times in 24 hours. If stomach pain or vomiting is increased by taking aspirin, the drug may be given rectally as a suppository.

As with almost all viral illnesses, there is no cure for chicken pox. Other remedies are soothing and comforting, can help relieve discomfort, and help the child to heal his/her body. There are a variety of treatments for the itch: a bath in a tubful of oatmeal suspension, in a baking-powder solution, or in water made cloudy with cornstarch is soothing. Calamine lotion or aloe will soothe the itch and help dry the pox. Ointments with benzocaine (a topical anesthetic) may be comforting but often result in allergic reactions. When there are many pox that are oozing fluid, soaks with aluminum acetate (Burow's Solution) will get the child past the oozing stage more quickly.

Temeril is a drug that acts on the central nervous system (actually as a kind of tranquilizer) and relieves itching. Ordinarily one would avoid treating the brain for a skin problem, unless simpler and safer remedies cannot make the child moderately comfortable. Another similar drug that relieves itch is the antihistamine Benadryl; it too should be used only if other measures are not helpful.

The discomforts of the mouth, esophagus, and stomach are best soothed by sips of cold, soothing, and nutritious drinks, such as a mixture of egg, milk, wheat germ, honey, and banana, and drinks mixed of yogurt, honey, and fruit or fruit juice. If vomiting or diarrhea is a significant problem one would have to alter the diet specifically to deal with the fluid loss (see sections on Vomiting and Diarrhea).

Cutting the child's nails short, keeping the hands clean, and covering the hands while the child sleeps will help keep scratching to a minimum. So will aspirin at bedtime, to give temporary relief from itch and help him/her to get to sleep. So will the offering of activities that occupy the hands while s/he is awake — cutting, pasting, coloring, and so on. Bathing the child every day with soap and water will help reduce the chance of bacterial infection. If pox do become infected with bacteria as a generalized complication, this problem can be treated by antibiotics taken by mouth or by injection, under the supervision of a professional.

Chicken-pox pneumonia does not need to be treated except with the usual home remedies for a respiratory infection: increased moisture in the air from a cool-mist vaporizer, honey-and-lemon or some similarly soothing cough remedy, and lots of fluids to drink. If the child's color becomes gray around the mouth, or if breathing is significantly difficult, treatment with oxygen in a hospital may be required. (Hospitals are very reluctant to admit a patient with chicken pox, since there are always patients who might become seriously ill with chicken pox and the disease is so very contagious).

Meningoencephalitis cannot be cured by any specific treatment. If signs and symptoms are sufficiently worrisome, admission to a hospital for observation may be advised. Ordinarily home care can reproduce hospital nursing care for this complication.

The period of contagiousness has passed when all the pox have dried. At this point the child can resume all social activities. If the illness has been severe, however, a few additional days of recuperation may be needed. As with all illnesses, this is a time for an especially nutritious diet. Children often do not eat well during illness, and may be comforted by sweets and other relatively nonnutritious food. While a few days of not eating will not hurt a well-nourished child, one would hope that whatever is eaten is maximally nutritious. If the child goes more than a day or so without a significant intake of nutritious food, one-a-day multivitamin tablets are probably helpful. Your ingenuity and your intimate knowledge of the child's food preferences will be exercised in inventing meals that are both tempting and promote healing.

## Collarbone (Clavicle) Fracture

The clavicle or collarbone is the slim bone that runs from the shoulder to the top of the breastbone. It is a bone that is frequently broken in children.

*Personal symptoms.* The child will refuse to move one arm, or will complain of pain when moving the arm. S/he may be able to remember falling on the arm or on the shoulder but often children cannot remember the fall because it was no more severe than other similar falls.

*Physical signs.* You will find no swelling or tenderness of the arm itself. There will be a point of tenderness as you press firmly with your fingers along the collarbone. You will want to have an X-ray taken to confirm that the clavicle has been broken.

*Remedies.* After the immediate remedies of aspirin for pain and comforting for the child, the treatment for a broken collarbone where the ends of the broken bone are lying close together (which is usually the case) is a bandage called a figure-of-eight, wrapped around the child's shoulders and upper back. Be sure to ask the doctor or nurse in the emergency room to show you how to wrap this bandage, in case you have to rewrap it in the next few days. As the bone heals there will be a lump of healing at the place where the bone was broken; you will be able to feel this lump for several months.

Don't forget to give the child an especially nutritious diet to assist in healing.

## Constipation

Constipation means hard stools that are difficult to pass and are passed infrequently. To identify constipation one must either be able to say that there is a change in the child's usual bowel habits, or that the child is experiencing significant distress, dysfunction, or disability.

*Personal symptoms.* For children, especially, constipation is a self-perpetuating cycle. Because the hard stools are painful to pass the child inhibits the body's signals to pass a stool, thus holding back the stool so that it becomes larger and harder. Sometimes, after constipation has gone on for several days, soft or even wet stool will leak out around the held-in hard stool, causing soiling or staining of diapers or underpants.

For a very few children, constipation is a perpetual and chronic condition from birth onward. These children have bowels that do not function properly; sometimes a surgical correction is necessary and helpful. For most children, constipation is a temporary condition.

Constipation can be initiated by factors in the child's diet. It can begin because the child's anus or rectum is sore and a normal stool is painful to pass. Or it can begin for a variety of reasons that are partly physical and partly emotional: not wanting to defecate at school or while traveling or at an unfamiliar home where the child is visiting, not wanting to interrupt play to use the toilet, conflict with a parent over who shall control the child's body, or the unwillingness or inability to make the effort to pass stool because of illness or depression.

An occasional hard or painful stool is usual for most of us, and requires no attention. Constipation that has lasted for two days should be remedied.

*Physical signs.* With older children, one must rely on the child's self-report to know about constipation. Habitual close questioning of the child about bowel habits may make the child feel that privacy is invaded, and make it less likely that the child will report painful, hard, or infrequent stools.

With children who are still in diapers, you do of course observe the frequency and consistency of stool every day. When the child is in the process of toilet training, or has just achieved this milestone, you must be very alert to signals from the child that s/he considers bowel movements personal business. This sense of privacy and autonomy must be respected, and yet you cannot help unless you are aware of a problem of constipation.

Hard and bulky stools that are unusual in color or consistency — stools that are pale or chalky in appearance, very oily, or that float in the toilet bowl — may indicate a digestive problem. The matter should be discussed with a professional.

You should examine the child's belly, feeling for masses of stool in the large bowel, backward from the rectum, up the left side of the belly, and across the top of the belly (see illustration 5). Examine the child's anus as well. A red and inflamed rash, a crack or fissure that becomes stretched and may streak the outside of a bulky stool with blood, or a tender and protruding hemorrhoid may explain the reason for the constipation.

*Other things you should know.* Diet is the most common cause of constipation in children, and dietary changes are the most usual solution to the problem. The second most frequent cause — and this is especially common for infants still in diapers — is a sore bottom that makes passage of stool painful.

Emotional causes for constipation become complicated by the child's need for privacy and self-regulation, by the embarrassment that most of us are taught to feel about toilet habits, and by the miseries that result from involuntary soiling of underpants. Fortunately, for older children the remedies for constipation can be regulated entirely by the child, if s/he so wishes.

*Remedies.* For children with sore bottoms, attention to the reason for the pain (with simultaneous softening of the stool to relieve the pain of passing stool) will quickly solve the problem. Rashes around the anus should be treated according to their appearance and cause, if that is known. A fissure will heal if it is protected during the passage of stool by a thick layer of petroleum jelly and if the stool is made so soft that it no longer causes stretching of the anus and cracking of the mucous membrane. Hemorrhoids (which are relatively rare before adolescence) are treated in the same way.

The stool can be softened in a matter of twelve hours by

a dose of mineral oil — one to two tablespoonsful for a small child, two to four tablespoonsful for an older child. Mix the mineral oil with a small amount of something tart and strong-flavored — concentrated lemonade or grapefruit juice works best — to mask the consistency as much as possible. If stools need to be kept soft for several days, regulate the amount of mineral oil in each dose according to the resulting consistency of stool — it should be soft and easy to pass but not watery or diarrheal. If the child takes more than one dose of mineral oil, a multivitamin tablet — containing vitamins A and D, the oil-soluble vitamins — should be given twelve hours after each dose of mineral oil, lest the oil wash these vitamins out of the bowel and the child become mildly vitamin deficient. Mineral oil is a temporary remedy, not to be used habitually.

If the impacted stool cannot be freed by mineral oil there will be leakage of soft oily stool around the impaction, with little muscular action of the bowel itself. Muscular action of the bowel can sometimes be stimulated by a simple glycerine suppository, sold in infant and adult sizes. Alternatively, a suppository can be carved out of any mild and unperfumed soap. The mechanical presence of the suppository can act as an irritant to cause the bowel to contract.

If unmedicated suppositories are not effective, one can give a chemical suppository that signals the muscles of the colon to contract. The drug is bisadocyl, sold as Dulcolax; it is a prescription drug.

Very rarely is the stool so bulky and so lodged in the bowel that it must be released with an enema. I feel very strongly that family members should not give enemas to constipated children. Even if a bowel problem does not begin as an emotion-laden condition, it quickly becomes one; children usually feel very violated by the administration of an enema. Ideally, an emergency-room nurse can do this calmly and kindly. If the nurse is disgruntled at performing this professional service (even though this is one situation when professional distance and objectivity is absolutely needed by families) one must decide whether the treatment the child receives at the hospital is worse than the distress experienced by this violation of the self by a parent.

If the constipation is not so chronic that one must soften the stool, the other remedies are all dietary. We know from international public-health surveys that bowel health seems to be directly related to nutritional habits. Specifically, diets high in undigestible food fiber seem to protect us not only against constipation but also against appendicitis, bowel cancer, and a disease of older age called diverticulitis. Dietary habits and preferences are strongly established in early childhood; one bout of constipation may be a helpful impetus to establish diet patterns that promote bowel health.

These are the recommendations to overcome or prevent constipation and to promote lifelong healthful bowel function:

- Foods high in undigestible fiber should be eaten in large amounts: bran, wheat germ, nuts and other unprocessed seeds and grains, and fruits and vegetables, especially eaten raw and especially with the skins and cores left to be eaten along with the meaty part of the fruit or vegetable. Think about ways of adding fruits and vegetables to every meal as well as snacks. Think about adding bran, especially, as frequently as you can to foods that you mix or bake — meat loaf, meatballs, casseroles, pancakes, muffins, bread.
- Foods with concentrated natural sugars — prunes, raisins, dates, and apricots — often have a specific laxative effect. Conversely, eating large amounts of refined white or brown sugar seems to be constipating for many persons.
- Yogurt is a specific bowel toner, known as such in many cultures. It is also a highly nutritious food, and is liked by many children when it is mixed with fresh-cut or dried fruit and with bran or wheat germ sprinkled on it. Resist the temptation to sweeten the yogurt unnecessarily; only those of us who have become addicted to sweets find the tartness of yogurt unpleasant.

This diet is, of course, nutritious and healthful in many ways. It usually straightens out constipation in a child very quickly. One should not, incidentally, give any over-the-counter or prescription laxatives to children except in the most extraordinary circumstances. All laxative preparations are habit-forming to some degree. Children do not need laxatives — except for the occasional dosage of a single Dulcolax suppository, as suggested above — to resolve problems of constipation, and they certainly do not need to be introduced to the use of addicting drugs.

It has been my impression that constipation has become an increasing problem for children in the last decade, despite the evident relaxation of mothers about the timing and pace of toilet training. If constipation cannot now be blamed on mothers' handling of the toilet-training issue, it seems to me that it must be due at least in part to our increasingly refined, processed, and sweetened diets. Adults as well as children can benefit from these dietary remedies for constipation.

## Convulsions

A convulsion is the expression of a massive electrical discharge in the cells of the central nervous system. A major motor (or grand mal) convulsion appears as repeated muscular contractions everywhere in the body, usually accompanied by unconsciousness. There are a variety of other kinds of convulsions, seen characteristically in the different types of epilepsy. Convulsions are also called seizures or fits.

*Personal symptoms.* The first convulsion that a child has is most likely to be the consequence of a fever, the first manifestation of epilepsy, an expression of poisoning, or the consequence of specific brain disease such as infection, tumor, or damage from trauma. Far and away the most common reason for a seizure in a child past infancy is fever. Febrile convulsions commonly occur, in susceptible children, when the temperature rises quickly from normal to some moderately high level at the beginning of an illness. Obviously, no one could foresee or prevent this kind of seizure at its first occurrence.

One wants also to think back over recent events when assessing a child who has had a convulsion. Could the child have gotten into some household substance or drug and become poisoned? Has there been a recent episode of head trauma? Has the child been coming down with an illness over the past few hours or days, especially an illness involving sleepiness or irritability, headache and stiff neck, suggesting an infection or inflammation of the central nervous system?

*Physical signs.* Convulsions are always emergencies, in the sense that one cannot do a complete health assessment and examination until the convulsion has come to an end. Most convulsions end quickly and spontaneously — although to the child's mother the episode seems to last for a frighteningly long time. It is tremendously important that the convulsion be observed and reported accurately. After you have done the immediate things to make the child comfortable, and have begun to make arrangements to bring the child to a professional (usually an emergency room), the most useful thing you can do is to pay close attention to what the child looks like. How did the convulsion begin? Was there a brief episode of staring or "absence"? Did the muscular movements begin in one particular part of the body and progress to other parts? Were both sides involved? Did the child's color ever become ashen in tone? Approximately how long did the convulsion last?

When the convulsion is over there will usually be an interval of sleepiness and lack of responsiveness. You will by now have made arrangements to transport the child. You should take the child's temperature and observe him/her closely for any evident signs of illness or injury. Don't forget to smell the child's breath as a clue to poisoning.

If your child has epilepsy or some other chronic condition that causes convulsions you will become very adept at first-aid treatment and at observing the events of the convulsion. Information from your observations of the convulsion can be very helpful in determining the appropriate treatment.

*Other things you should know.* Convulsions are frightening events for mothers and also for other observers. No one is cool, calm, and collected in the face of a first convulsion in a loved one. It takes lengthy training as a professional to be able to make detailed and accurate observations of convulsions. As the child's mother, you will do well to keep your head, make some appropriate first-aid gestures, and remember some of what you saw. After the convulsion is over (unless the child has a chronic tendency to repeated convulsions) you will need the help of a professional to determine the cause of the convulsion and the treatment, if any.

Remember that most convulsions are due to fever, and most children with a febrile convulsion never have another one. Many other causes of convulsions are treatable. One convulsion does not mean that the child has a serious or life-threatening disease or will have a lifelong tendency to repeated convulsions.

Some children hold their breath in a temper tantrum. The breath-holding causes a lack of oxygen in the brain. If the child continues for long enough, facial color will become ashen, s/he will become unconscious, and may twitch the arms and legs. Of course, as soon as s/he is unconscious any willful breath-holding will stop. S/he will not be hurt by this maneuver, although it is more than a little embarrassing when done in a public place. Like all forms of temper tantrums, this is best dealt with by ignoring. That is, you need to check that s/he has not been hurt by falling, but you must be careful not to give the child the message that this behavior is a good way for him/her to get what s/he wants. You can avert breath-holding spells sometimes by anticipating the child's frustrations and providing distraction, or you can comfort the child in a variety of ways after the fact, but you do not want to show that this behavior will help the child make his/her way in the world.

Convulsions themselves are rarely harmful to a child. If s/he has a respiratory infection or chokes on respiratory secretions so that facial color becomes gray, s/he may not be getting enough oxygen to the brain. In a child, even this occurrence rarely causes any permanent damage, but this gray color (called cyanosis) is a reason to get the child as quickly as possible to a place that has oxygen.

*Remedies.* The first and most important step in caring for a child who is having a convulsion is to turn the child to one side, preferably with the head low, to allow the drainage of secretions from the mouth and throat. This maneuver will usually prevent the problem of lack of oxygen. Loosen the child's clothes and be sure that s/he will not be injured by falling or bumping against objects. Do not try to force the jaws apart to put some object in the mouth; this is rarely successful and can cause hurt.

Long-term remedies for convulsions depend on the cause. Usually there is no recommended treatment for a child who has had one febrile convulsion. Since the fit is likely to occur at the beginning of an illness when the temperature is rising rapidly, there is no way to predict and treat in advance of a seizure.

When a child has had two febrile convulsions it is usually recommended that the child be given phenobarbital, an anticonvulsive medication, every day until the age of 6 or so. Since this medicine is a sedative, one does not want to give it unnecessarily and risk dulling the child's learning capacities. It is given only when the possibility of repeated convulsions seems high, and only because each successive convulsion seems to predispose the child to more convulsions, rather like wearing down a path for the electrical impulses to travel along.

There are many medicines for epilepsy. Most children can be kept seizure-free with some combination of drugs. Many of the anticonvulsant drugs have significant undesirable side effects; they should only be prescribed by physicians with experience in treating this sort of childhood illness.

## Cough

A cough is sudden expulsion of air from the lungs, with sufficient force to make noise. Sometimes this rapid high air pressure clears the breathing tubes of phlegm and other material.

*Personal symptoms.* A cough that is more than occasional is a signal of some kind of respiratory difficulty. That difficulty may be located as high as the juncture of the nose and throat, or it may be at the bottom reaches of the lungs.

Coughs can also be an expression of nervous tension. In this case no signs or symptoms of illness or injury can be found, the cough will appear to be worse when emotional stress is heightened, and will go away when the child's need for it — the basis of the tension and stress — is soothed.

A cough may reflect an allergic condition, with an excessive production of respiratory secretions. These secretions may be very wet and juicy, as in the case of postnasal drip. In this condition excessive secretions from the mucous membranes of the nose run backward into the throat — especially while the child is asleep — and result in a cough that clears the secretions from the area of the throat at and above the tongue. An allergic cough may also indicate dry, tacky, bronchial secretions, as in asthma; the cough is frequent and nonproductive because the sticky secretions do not move easily out of the breathing tubes.

A cough may reflect infection and the need to clear the airway of the material that accumulates as a consequence of the infection: excessive mucous mixed with the infecting agent (usually a virus or bacteria) and the substances that the body mobilizes to combat the infection, such as blood cells, antibodies, and so on. These are common locations for infection:

- At the back of the throat — tonsillitis (unless the tonsils have been removed) or pharyngitis.
- At the epiglottis, the fleshy valve that covers the windpipe when we swallow. Infection here gives symptoms of croup and a short, barky cough.
- In the area from the voice box down through the main central breathing tube or bronchus — laryngotracheobronchitis. Infection here can also cause symptoms of croup; when the larynx is involved the voice may be hoarse.
- In the large and medium-sized breathing tubes — bronchitis.
- In the smallest breathing tubes — bronchiolitis.
- In the lung tissue that lies at the end of each tiny breathing tube — pneumonia. Pneumonia may be generalized, in every area of the lungs, or it may be confined to one lobe on one side, the area connected to one medium-sized breathing tube and its smaller branches.

This list suggests greater precision in localizing the area of infection than is often possible. Even with an X-ray, only some direct signs of infection can be seen; other infected areas may not appear abnormal on the X-ray.

A foreign object may have been inhaled and become stuck in one of the breathing tubes. Cough can also result from the drying of respiratory secretions. This comes about when the air breathed is very dry, as in the winter in temperate climates when house heat is on.

In considering the reason for your child's cough, you should think about the possibility of an allergic reaction; exposure — known or unknown — to infections; and the possibility of an inhaled foreign body. Look for other symptoms of illness — complaint of pain, for instance. Consider the degree of difficulty that your child is having in breathing, and the overall degree of illness shown by irritability, sleepiness, poor appetite, inability to play, and so on.

*Physical signs.* The vital signs of temperature and respiratory rate will help you decide about the presence of bacterial infection (which is likely to give a moderate to high fever) or viral infection (which is likely to give a low to moderate fever), and about the degree of dysfunction of the breathing system. Consider the timing and the character of the cough.

The cough of hay fever or nasal allergy, with postnasal drip, usually occurs in the night and on arising in the morning. It is a mildly productive cough — you can hear that some material is being moved as the child coughs. Most children swallow the material that they bring to the throat by coughing.

The cough of asthma is dry and initially nonproductive. As treatment proceeds and the dry mucous loosens, the cough should become moderately productive.

The cough of a sore throat is tickly, frequent, short, and nonproductive. It is primarily a reflex cough and serves no useful purpose.

Coughs that result from infections in the lower respiratory tract may be nonproductive at the beginning of an illness. But there is always, with an infection, some production of a mixture of cells and mucous. This material needs to be cleared out of the respiratory tract, and the cough is therefore a necessary part of the healing. A cough is a helpful reflex and serves an important purpose.

One would like to be able to discover the reason for the cough. Only certain things can be known about the respiratory tract by examination, however. One searches for this information, couples it with what is known about exposure to infections, the child's past history of wellness and illness, and current complaints, and makes an informed guess about the reason for the cough. Doctors and nurses do just this.

Examine the nose for mucous production. Look at the throat for signs of inflammation. Feel the nodes of the neck for enlargement and tenderness. Check the ears.

Observe the pattern of breathing, the rate, any sign of prolongation of the breathing-in phase (croup) or of the breathing-out phase (asthma). When breathing is labored, the accessory muscles of respiration — muscles that can increase the respiratory effort — can be seen in action. The nostrils flare and the spaces between the ribs depress with each inspiration. Note the child's color — an ashen look around the mouth suggests that the child is not getting enough oxygen. Listen with the stethoscope. You will have familiarized yourself with the breathing sounds your child makes when well, and can recognize changes associated with the cough. You may hear:

- Rhonchi, noisy, loose rattling sounds, heard best in the upper central part of the back and front of the chest. These sounds usually clear entirely or to a major degree when the child coughs. The sounds reflect the presence of loose mucous and other material in the central breathing tube and its largest branches; they may even be transmitted from higher in the respiratory apparatus. They signify material in the breathing apparatus that is not ordinarily there, and explain the need for cough. They rarely signify serious disease, themselves. They are common with viral colds and allergies, and with pharyngitis.

- Wheezes, which are fine, whistling sounds heard characteristically with expiration (breathing out) in asthma, but also sometimes heard in both the in and out phases of breathing. These sounds reflect excess material in the middle-sized and small breathing tubes, the smallest of which are called bronchioles. Wheezes do not clear completely with coughing, and indicate some degree of bronchitis.

- Rales, which are the quietest sounds of all. They come from the movement of excess material in the tiny air sacs at the very periphery of the lungs, the sacs that lie beyond the bronchioles, the spaces where fresh oxygen is exchanged for waste gases. Rales sound like tissue paper crackling, or like the quiet noise of fingers being rubbed together. Presumably they come from the breaking of tiny bubbles of fluid in the elastic sacs as the sacs expand and contract. The presence of rales indicates pneumonia, which is inflammation or infection of the lung tissue itself.
- No sound at all in an area in which there are breath sounds on the other side of the chest. This indicates that air is not moving in that space — because of a pneumonia or some other space-occupying process, or because of an obstructing foreign body.

*Remedies.* Coughs are treated in two stages. First, it must be decided whether *any* remedy is needed or will be helpful for the condition that underlies the cough. Second, there are remedies that can be given for the symptom of cough itself.

It would make no sense to treat the *cough* caused by a foreign object stuck in a breathing tube. The remedy must remove the foreign object. Similarly, if the cough is the result of a bacterial infection — of the throat, the epiglottis, the bronchi, or the lungs — there are remedies that help to overcome bacterial infections and they should be chosen first. A decision about the probable bacterial origin of a cough will depend on signs of infection in other respiratory areas (throat, ears, lymph nodes); the amount of fever, with bacterial infections usually causing a higher temperature than viral infections (there are notable exceptions); the count and pattern of white blood cells, since the body puts forth different kinds of cells to combat bacterial and viral infections; and, in some instances, the picture of the infection seen on X-ray. If the infection seems to be bacterial and of a serious nature an antibiotic will be recommended.

If there seems to be infection and it is thought that the infection is viral, remedies will be directed only to symptoms and will support self-healing. If the child has been in contact

with others with a similar cough and those others have recovered easily with no specific remedy being given, it is likely
that the child will follow a similar course.

There are a variety of remedies for cough:

- Drinking extra fluids of any kind will tend to loosen the
  secretions that are being coughed; even if the secretions
  are already loose, extra fluids will not harm and may help.
- A cool-mist vaporizer will bring moisture directly into the
  breathing apparatus, tending both to loosen the secretions
  and to soothe a cough that is primarily irritative.
- Direct local soothing: honey and lemon juice, plain or
  mixed with a little hot water, accomplishes this.
- Remedies that act on the brain: aspirin has a general sedative effect, and so does a little whiskey, which can be
  mixed with the honey and lemon. Codeine and dextro-
  methorphan act more directly on the cough center in the
  brain.
- Expectorant and mucolytic drugs loosen the secretions:
  examples are lemon juice, ginger, and cayenne pepper,
  which increase secretions in the stomach and also in the
  respiratory tree by a kind of sympathetic action, and glyc-
  eryl guaiacolate and ipecac, which are found in commercial cough preparations.
- Bronchodilators like theophylline and epinephrine make
  the breathing tubes relax and open.
- Antihistamines can dry respiratory secretions, act as bronchodilators, and act as central nervous system sedatives.

The decision about how to treat a cough will depend on
your observations of the child. Productive coughing is part of
the healing mechanism. If the cough is not very productive,
you may want to try to loosen the secretions. If the cough
disturbs sleep or interferes with the child's talking or playing,
it should be sedated. If the child coughs in his sleep but sleeps
soundly, this is not a reason for sedation. If the cough is so
juicy that the child chokes, some drying may be in order. If
wheezing is handicapping, bronchodilators may be given.

Most coughs need no commercial remedy. Honey and
lemon and herbal teas, extra fluids to drink and extra moisture

in the room air are usually all that is needed to soothe and
help the child cough what needs to be coughed.


## Cradle Cap and Infant Seborrhea

Seborrhea is a greasy, scaly rash that is caused by an inefficient
function of the glands of the skin that produce sebum, a lubri-
cating substance.

*Personal Symptoms.* In infants — in whom this rash is
common — the red, rough appearance is seen in the first few
days or weeks after birth; most commonly it is noticed at the
age of 2 or 3 weeks. The rash on the face, trunk, and arms
disappears two or three months later; the rash on the scalp
(cradle cap) may persist until the age of 3 or 4. For some
individuals, this rash reappears throughout life; on the scalp,
in later years, the rash is called dandruff. It causes no discomfort except, occasionally in older persons, an itch.

*Physical signs.* The rash is most commonly seen on the
forehead, around the mouth and on the chin, on the trunk and
upper arms; sometimes it covers most of the body. On the body
it appears as small, slightly raised bumps, which may look red
and inflamed. It has a slightly greasy feel. On the scalp it
appears as flat, greasy scales, which pile up to make a layer or
plaque that is yellow or gray.

*Other things you should know.* The rash of seborrhea is
common in infants because their skin is immature; the glands
that produce sebum are not working very efficiently. When the
rash appears on the skin at later ages it probably also means
that the glands do not work efficiently, at least off and on, for
that person. For infants, at least, it should not be considered
a disease; the primary reason to treat it is because it is a little
unsightly and thus disturbing to mothers.

If there are small, raised, yellowish bumps the rash of
seborrhea may have become infected with bacteria, and some
antibiotic ointment may be helpful. Rashes in the diaper area
(or rashes that begin in the diaper area and spread to other
parts of the body) are likely to be something other than
seborrhea.

*Remedies.* Sometimes the rash is most prominent on one side if the baby always sleeps on one side; try turning the child or encouraging him/her to sleep on the other side by hanging something bright to look at on one side of the crib.

For a seborrheic rash on the skin, a simple steroid ointment will decrease the inflammation and often make the rash go away altogether. There are a variety of steroid ointments marketed. Hydrocortisone cream or lotion (one percent) is a common and relatively inexpensive preparation — although all steroid preparations are costly, and all are available only by prescription. Apply it very thinly, three or four times a day, only so often as is needed to keep the rash minimized.

For seborrhea of the scalp, rub some simple oil (mineral oil, baby oil, or olive oil) into the baby's scalp an hour or two before shampoo time. Shampoo with a mild soap, washing and rinsing well enough to remove the oil. Then take a fine comb and scrub lightly on the scales, removing by combing all that will easily loosen. For some children, this kind of a shampoo-and-grooming routine will need to be done off and on for years.

## Croup

Croup is a respiratory difficulty characterized by labored inspiration, with a stridor (a noisy rasp) heard each time the child breathes in.

*Personal symptoms.* Some children are particularly prone to croup, while others never get croupy. Croupiness can start as early as the first year of life, but is usually outgrown in adolescence. Some children get croupy almost every time they have a respiratory infection. These children usually have, in addition to inspiratory stridor, a harsh and barky cough and some hoarseness as part of the illness.

There are some viruses and one bacteria that specifically cause croupy breathing, even in children who do not ordinarily have croup. The viral infections do not have specific remedies, and are treated as any episode of croup is treated — with symptomatic and supportive measures. The bacterial infection — caused by *Haemophilus influenza* — can be treated specifically with antibiotics, the most common remedy now being the penicillin derivative ampicillin.

A child with croup can feel very panicky, especially if s/he awakens from a sound sleep with croup. The child may feel that s/he will not be able to take another breath. A mother gets panicky, too, when she sees the child so alarmed. Becoming more familiar with croup will make you more confident that you can help the child.

Croup usually starts very suddenly. You may have been able to predict that it was going to come, from the child's past history and from the child's condition at bedtime. Croup can usually be turned off just as suddenly.

*Physical signs.* Croup is an emergency, and therefore remedies must begin at once. Assessment of the child's condition must wait until the severity of the respiratory distress has eased. A more thorough examination can be done after the child's croup has eased.

When the child has first awakened and your immediate concern is to ease the croup, you will do no more assessment than to estimate body temperature by feeling the forehead, and observe the breathing for a few minutes to notice the rate of respiration, the degree of stridor, and the color around the mouth, noting pallor or an ashen color that signifies oxygen lack. If the child does look oxygen-deficient, you will immediately arrange to take the child to an emergency room — although in the process of getting the child ready s/he may improve, and you can then proceed with home remedies.

*Remedies.* There are three principal home remedies that are effective in turning off a croup of sudden onset: taking the child to a space with very humid air to breathe; taking the child to very cold air to breathe; and making the child vomit. If your child is croupy — has recurrent episodes of croup — you will learn what is most effective.

Here is a step-by-step outline for treating a child with croup:

- Note quickly the child's general condition — fever, rate of breathing, color, ear-pulling or other indication of earache, and degree of cough. Does s/he seem distracted or unresponsive, or is s/he trying to talk spontaneously? Hold the child and talk to him/her comfortingly as you do this.

- If your soothing has not aided the child in breathing more easily, you will want to decide whether to call someone else to assist you — another adult in the house, an older child, a relative, friend, or neighbor.
- Give the child a dose of aspirin (or aspirin substitute), both for fever and for its sedative effect.
- Turn on all the faucets in the bathroom to as hot a setting as possible, and make a comfortable place in the bathroom for you and the child to sit; bring a story to read.
- Bring a favorite drink for the child to sip; ask the child what s/he wants — something cold or something hot?
- Think what else will help the child to relax. A rocking chair? A lullaby? A back rub?
- You will ordinarily wait a half hour — the time it takes for aspirin to have an effect — to see if this regimen is going to turn off the croup. You are aiming for a decrease in the child's panic and a decrease in the laboring of breathing, a relaxation so that s/he can go to sleep. The noisiness of breathing may remain, along with a barky cough.
- If the cough is persistent and fatiguing for the child, there are two remedies that are usually helpful. The first is a teaspoonful of honey mixed with lemon juice, diluted with a very small amount of hot water. The second is a commercial cough remedy that you will have on hand if your child tends to be croupy. Ipsatol (plain, without sedative) is almost a specific remedy for a croupy, barky cough.
- If the child is worsening — looking more gray, becoming more silent, more sleepy or agitated, or seeming more panicky about the breathing difficulty — you will want to go to a hospital emergency room. Depending on your relationship with your doctor and on your experience with the hospital, you may want to call ahead to say that you are on your way with your child. Because of the breathing difficulty, you will want to go to a place where oxygen can be given to the child immediately, if necessary; this is not

usually true in a doctor's office. The child may also need to have blood tests done. Breathing difficulties can cause a change in the balance of gases and salts that are dissolved in the blood. You should understand also that if you go to an emergency room with a croupy child the primary question for the examining doctor will be whether the child should be admitted to the hospital, for observation if not for treatment.

- Whether you are headed for the hospital or just waiting a little longer to see whether the child improves spontaneously, the next step is to bring the child into cool air to breathe. That means going outside if the outside temperature is cooler than the temperature inside the house. Standing in front of an open refrigerator may have the same effect. Sudden exposure to cool air often stops croupiness quite dramatically. If you are on your way to the hospital and have notified the doctor or the emergency room that you are coming, you may find that by the time you get there the crisis is over and the child's breathing is easy again. Doctors who take care of children will have experienced this before, although they may react with irritation and assume that you made a precipitous and thoughtless decision to come to the hospital. You will know differently.

- One additional method for stopping croup that works for some children is worth trying at home, unless you decide that you need immediate professional consultation. Use your finger to gag the child. This will make him/her vomit.

- If despite all these remedies the child is not better (even if s/he is not significantly worse), if there is high fever, or if you feel that the child is too agitated to sleep, you will want to go to the hospital. There a decision will be made about hospitalization for observation. Except for oxygen administration, hospital nurses can do no more to provide an instant cure for croup than you can at home. In addition, a decision will be made about the use of an antibiotic, if the croup seems to be of bacterial origin.

- If your remedies have made the child better, proceed with

the usual physical examination. Measure the respiratory rate and temperature. Listen to the breathing with a stethoscope, checking for the noises of bronchitis. Examine ears and throat, and feel the lymph nodes of the neck; flex the neck forward to be sure it is supple. Examine the skin for rashes.

Usually, croup that is caused by a virus infection begins to be much better in about 24 hours. If after 24 hours the croupy spells are as severe as they were in the beginning — even if they are controllable by your home remedies — you will want to have the child seen by a professional.

### Diaper Rash

Rashes that begin in the diaper area are most commonly caused by contact of the skin with some irritating substance, or by a common skin fungus called monilia.

*Personal symptoms.* Diaper rashes can begin as a faint redness and become progressively more inflamed, or can appear full-blown within a few hours' time. Only rarely do babies seem to be bothered by diaper rashes; older babies may act as if the rash were itchy, and sometimes if the rash is open and oozing an infant may be irritable as if the rash area were painful.

*Physical signs.* A diaper rash or contact rash is usually red and flat, with margins that fade into normal-appearing skin. At first there is no rash within the folds of skin in the groin and the upper legs.

A monilial rash usually has fairly distinct edges, slightly raised. There may be smaller patches of rash outside the edges of the central rash. This rash usually begins within the skin folds.

If there is an additional infection with bacteria, the rash can have small raised yellow blisters, called pustules.

*Other things you should know.* Contact rashes can be caused by urine, as when the diaper is changed infrequently. This is especially likely to occur when you are traveling or visiting and cannot find opportunities for diaper changes. It happens also when the baby is older, makes more concentrated urine, and naps for a long time or sleeps through the whole night.

Stool can also be irritating on contact. This is likely to be true when the child has a diarrhea. It also happens when the baby is teething and is making extra saliva; there is a substance in saliva at these times that can be very irritating to skin. The contact rash from the stool of a teething baby may appear in the space of a single nap, and can look flaming red like a slapped area or a burn.

Some babies get a red contact rash from disposable diapers. Some also react to laundry preparations, especially to detergents if the diapers are not well rinsed. Occasionally some food that the baby has eaten or that a nursing mother has eaten will come through in the stool and cause a contact rash.

Monilia is a fungus that most of us carry on our skins. Only some people are susceptible to a skin rash from monilia. It may be the immaturity of babies' skin that makes them susceptible.

Bacteria, also, are present on our skin at all times. Bacteria usually cause festering when there are breaks in the surface of the skin, even very tiny breaks that are difficult to notice.

*Remedies.* If the rash appears to be a contact rash, think of the most likely causes and try to remedy them: change diapers more frequently, consider changing the way you do the laundry, think about foods that you or the baby ate before the rash appeared. Try using cloth instead of disposable diapers.

The most helpful remedy for a contact rash is to leave the skin exposed to air — and, if weather permits, to sunlight. Leave the diapers off as much as you practically can.

When the baby must be diapered, apply some protective ointment, using a thick layer. Useful protective ointments are those made with petroleum jelly (Vasoline or A and D), and those made with zinc oxide (Desitin or Peri-Anal).

Very occasionally, if the inflammation is marked and there seems to be no infection, a steroid ointment like hydrocortisone 1% (available on a prescription) is helpful.

If the rash appears to be monilial, there are special prescription ointments that will combat the fungus; two commonly used brands are Mycostatin and Sporostacin. These should be used when the baby is diapered; again, exposure to light and air will give the skin a chance to heal. Think also about possible irritants that might have given the fungus a chance to invade the skin and to grow. Treat the cause of the contact dermatitis, if you have an idea what that might be.

If there is bacterial infection it will be helpful to bathe the diaper area for a few days with an antibacterial soap like pHisoderm, pHisohex, or Betadyne — the latter two are prescription drugs. Leaving the diapers off is also helpful for a bacterial infection. Be sure to wash your own hands well after you have handled the baby.

## Diarrhea

Diarrhea is the frequent passage of watery stools.

*Personal symptoms.* Diarrhea is commonly caused by infections of the gastrointestinal tract; ingestion of spoiled food; by infections in other parts of the body, such as ear infections and urinary-tract infections; by drugs, especially anitbiotics; and by a variety of specific diseases of bowel dysfunction. Swallowing excessive mucous, as happens with a cough or with teething, can also cause loose stools. One or two loose stools is not ordinarily considered diarrhea, but if the stools are voluminous and especially if the child is an infant even diarrhea of brief duration should be taken very seriously.

A first determination is to consider whether the diarrhea might be due to a condition of some body part other than the bowel. Might the child be coming down with an upper-respiratory infection? Is s/he pulling at the ears or acting as if s/he has an earache? Is there any sign of an infection of the urinary tract? Has a by-mouth antibiotic been given recently? If the child is an infant, has the nursing mother's diet changed in the last few days? What new foods have recently been introduced? Remembering that infants may show minimal or unexpected signs of ordinary illnesses, are there *any* indications of disease such as crankiness or irritability, excessive sleepiness, or refusal to nurse or to eat solid foods?

*Physical signs.* Examination of the child with diarrhea should include a search for causes of the diarrhea in other areas of the body. Think about ear infections, throat infections, rashes, stiff neck and enlarged lymph nodes, and lung problems. Examination of the belly will include the consideration of the possibility of bowel obstruction, which sometimes produces small diarrheal stools of mucous and blood. You should weigh a child with serious diarrhea daily. (See section on vomiting for the signs of dehydration.)

*Remedies.* Diarrhea alone is treated in a somewhat different fashion than diarrhea that occurs with vomiting. When diarrhea is the only symptom, the first consideration is to treat any cause of the diarrhea apart from the bowel. That is, infections elsewhere in the body — such as ear infections or urinary-tract infections — should be treated with specific antibiotics.

The diarrhea itself is treated by putting the bowel to rest, feeding only simple, clear liquids in large enough quantities to replace the fluids lost from the bowel. Simple, clear liquids are mixtures of water, salts, and carbohydrates. They are called "clear" because they are usually somewhat transparent. Examples are diluted fruit juices, popsicles and jellied solids made from fruit juice, sherbet made without milk, weak broth, and herbal teas. A well-nourished child can get along without solid food for 24 to 48 hours, and the bowel at rest will heal itself if the reason for the diarrhea is located within the bowel.

It is best not to treat a child with diarrhea with paregoric or other opiumlike drugs. Lomotil, an antidiarrheal drug sometimes given to adults, should rarely be used for children.

There is a primitive body reflex, seen almost always in. infants, that stimulates the bowel to evacuate whenever anything enters the stomach. This reflex often is reactivated when there is diarrhea, even if the child is long past infancy, so that whenever the child drinks (or eats) the bowel is stimulated to produce another stool. For this reason, diarrhea should be treated by giving few feedings of relatively large amounts of fluid.

Vomiting is treated in exactly the opposite way from diarrhea, by giving frequent feedings of small amounts of clear liquids. When vomiting and diarrhea occur together, one must estimate which symptom is causing the larger fluid loss, and feed at first in a manner designed to get rid of that symptom. Ordinarily it is easier to get rid of the vomiting first, by feeding in small amounts frequently. When the vomiting has come to an end, one can increase the volume of feedings and decrease their frequency to treat the diarrhea. If, on the other hand, the vomiting is infrequent and in small amounts from the beginning and the diarrhea is the major source of loss of body fluids, one should begin by treating the diarrhea.

Usually, 24 hours of putting the bowel to rest by feeding diluted clear liquids will end a diarrhea. Feedings of solids should be resumed gradually, avoiding in the beginning foods containing indigestible fiber and fatty foods. When foodstuffs are not being absorbed properly, it is important to stop feeding the offending foods. Good foods for the first feedings after a clear liquid diet include cooked carrots, soft meats with a low fat content such as chicken and veal, dry bread or toast and soda crackers, clear noodle soup, scraped apple and banana. Yogurt, which always has some effect as a bowel toner, is also a good starter food.

If the diarrhea has resulted from the feeding of a by-mouth antibiotic, it probably reflects an overgrowth in the bowel of bacteria or fungi that are usually present in low concentration. This is a consequence of the killing by the antibiotic of the useful bacteria that ordinarily inhabit the bowel. The lost bacteria can most quickly be replaced by feeding yogurt in large amounts, otherwise following the clear liquid diet. If this is not successful, or if the child will not eat yogurt, there are granules called Lactinex that contain the same friendly bowel bacteria that yogurt contains. If one is near the end of a course of antibiotics, or if the diarrhea can be controlled by yogurt or by Lactinex, one should continue to give the antibiotic to help heal the condition for which it was originally recommended. If the diarrhea gets out of hand, it may be necessary to give the antibiotic by injection or to prescribe a different antibiotic.

For small infants, milk is too necessary a food to be gone without for more than about 12 hours. Breast-fed babies should be offered alternate feedings of breast milk and diluted juice or herbal tea with honey, after a period of 12 hours of clear-liquid feedings. Babies who are accustomed to drinking pre-pared commercial formula should be offered their regular for-mula, prepared to full strength and then diluted half-and-half with water. Babies who are drinking cows' milk — evaported, skim, or whole — should be offered skim milk, brought to a boil to increase the digestibility of the protein and then diluted half-and-half with water. Never feed a baby boiled skim milk without diluting it with water *after* it has boiled; otherwise the concentration of salt in the milk can reach dangerous levels.

If the diarrhea persists and there is still no sign of an explanatory cause in some illness affecting another part of the body, one should seek professional consultation for a thorough examination and laboratory tests. A urinary-tract infection, which may cause no other symptoms, will be suspected.

Timing of consultation with a professional will vary greatly with diarrheas in children. If stools are frequent and loose, the treatment — putting the bowel at rest with an ample intake of clear liquids — may also serve to maintain the child in an even metabolic state. If there are no other severe com-plaints and no apparent signs of causative disease, no harm is done in waiting hours or days for the treatment to work and the diarrhea to subside. If, on the other hand, the stools are explosive, watery, and voluminous, if the child is very young and therefore at a high risk of dehydration, if there are symp-toms or signs of some illness other than simple bowel dys-function, or if the child acts worrisomely ill with crankiness, sleepiness, or high fever, then you will want to consult a professional much earlier in the disease.

Once a child begins with a diarrhea the loose and frequent stools may continue on for weeks. There may not be enough fluid loss to cause a problem but there will be all the bother of diarrhea. The younger the child the more this is likely to be true; it is as if the bowel has to relearn normal function, and this is difficult. Needed nutrition is always lost with diarrhea:

stools pass through the bowel quickly and foodstuffs fail to be absorbed into the bloodstream. If this happens you will want to ask a professional to review the situation, even though by this time the child may not seem at all ill. There are relatively uncommon causes for diarrhea that can be discovered by laboratory tests, causes such as intestinal parasites, that need to be considered and treated if possible.

Diarrheal disease is very common in childhood. The great majority of diarrheas are simple and self-limited, and with appropriate care at home come to an end fairly quickly.

**Ear Wax**

Ear wax (also called cerumen) is a yellow or brown substance secreted by glands in the external ear canal; it varies in texture from dry and tenaciously sticky, to liquid and somewhat oily. It functions to trap any small particle that enters the ear canal. Small hairs lining the ear canal beat rhythmically to move the wax toward the external opening of the canal and thus keep the canal (and the eardrum at the back of the canal) cleared of small objects and particles. Ear wax can become impacted, massed, in front of the eardrum.

*Personal symptoms.* When ear wax is packed against the eardrum, you may become aware that your child is not hearing as well as s/he usually does. Or s/he may complain that one or both ears seem blocked, and that it is harder than usual to hear. Never rely on the child's report about hearing acuity, for s/he may not realize that hearing acuity is diminished. Note how loudly s/he is speaking, whether s/he turns the TV or radio to a volume louder than usual, and whether s/he can hear you when you offer something inviting by whispering behind his/her back. S/he might also complain if there is impacted ear wax that the ears feel full or itchy.

The most common cause of impacted ear wax is putting something into the ear canal. The most usual reason to put some implement — like a Q-tip — into the ear canal is to clean out ear wax. Not only is there a risk of scratching the sides of the ear canal (a very painful accident) by this procedure, but

most commonly the implement only succeeds in removing a
small amount of the ear wax loose in the canal, forcing the rest
up against the eardrum.

We do seem to have a kind of fetish about ear wax. Not
long ago I worked on a mobile medical van that brought medical services to "street kids," many of them runaways. They
did not have enough food, no regular place to sleep, no place
to bathe, and no fresh clothes to change into. In short, they
were dirty and often smelly, although these were never issues
for discussion (except for sympathy), since the youngsters usually also had significant illness or injury problems that brought
them to the medical van. They themselves rarely remarked on
their state of dishevelment — perhaps because teenagers feel
relatively comfortable to be that way — but they almost invar-
iably commented on their ear wax. As I prepared to examine
their ears, they would say apologetically, "I'm sorry, I don't
think I cleaned out my ears today." Either their mothers had
done a good job of teaching them that cleaning out one's ear
canals was an important part of daily hygiene, or doctors in
their past experience had been annoyed to look into their ear
canals and find them full of wax.

*Physical signs.* In fact, it is in most cases possible to examine the eardrums by looking around the wax that lies along
the sides of the canal. Occasionally, and very carefully, one
might remove a small bit of wax with a cerumen spoon in
order to see the entire surface of the eardrum. In most cases,
however, one can get a view of the eardrum using a smaller or
larger tip for the otoscope, and by pulling gently on the external ear to change the direction of the canal.

When ear wax is packed solidly against the eardrum you
cannot see the drum at all. This is almost always the result of
implements having been pushed down into the ear canal. A
few rare individuals have ear wax so tenaciously sticky that it
cannot be completely moved out of the ear canals by the action
of the tiny hairs.

If there is a suspicion of hearing loss, one should never
proceed with a hearing test (an audiogram) without ascertain-
ing that the eardrums are not blocked by wax. This can be
accomplished by consulting with a professional, or it can be

done at home if you have access to an otoscope and are practiced in using it.

*Remedies.* The first remedy is preventive — don't stick
implements into the ear canal. When wax does become impacted, consider first whether there has been any recent episode of drainage — of blood, pus, or clear fluid — from the ear
canal. If this is true you will not want to do anything about ear
wax until a professional has examined the eardrums to be sure
that they are intact.

The remedy for impacted ear wax is very simple. Mix
hydrogen peroxide half-and-half with water and flood the ear
canal with this mixture, using an eyedropper. Have the child
hold the head to one side for as long as possible or comfortable — never very long for a toddler — and then let the
liquid run out, carrying some dissolved wax with it. Repeat
this procedure for the other ear. The most stubbornly impacted
wax will be dissolved in four or five once-a-day repeats of this
procedure. Often only a single treatment will do the trick.

Ear wax can also be washed out using an electrical implement called a Water-Pik. This is somewhat more difficult to
accomplish, since plain water will not soften or dissolve the
wax. If the water pressure is too high, the stream of water will
hurt as it hits the eardrum.

Some people have such dry ear wax that they complain of
itchy ears. Scratching with any implement may injure the
canals or pack ear wax. Burow's Solution (aluminum acetate)
can be bought in inexpensive tablet form as Domeboro tablets
and mixed, one tablet to a quart of water. Use a bit of cotton
or gauze for a wick and keep the wick moist with the solution,
changing the wick every day. This is also a useful treatment
for an infection of the ear canal (swimmer's ear, or otitis ex-
terna), which is the other common cause of itching in the ear
canal.

## Fever

Fever is body temperature higher than normal, or average,
body temperature: 36.4°C/97.6°F measured in the armpit,
37°C/98.6°F measured by mouth, or 37.6°C/99.6°F measured by

rectum. To know whether a child has an elevated body temperature, you should ideally know what that child's usual body temperature is at different times of the day.

*Personal symptoms.* A child with a fever may look hot and flushed and complain of feeling hot, or s/he may look pale, have goosebumps, and complain of chills. There is no regular correspondence between the amount of fever, the degree of distress that the child experiences, and the severity of the illness. A severe infection may cause only a small elevation of temperature. Conversely, a child may feel quite ill, have only a little fever, and have a mild illness. At some point in the fever rise — this point differs for different children — the child will experience some discomfort from the fever itself. That distress may range from feeling warm, to shivering, to feeling sleepy, to irritability and feeling jittery.

Some children convulse with a fever. These children fall into two groups. Children who are seizure-prone (who have seizures on other occasions) may have seizures when they have a fever, even a low-grade fever. Other children have febrile seizures. This happens only when there is a moderate to high elevation of body temperature and usually when body temperature rises very quickly from normal to a high level. This happens most frequently at the beginning of an illness; the child seems fine one moment, and then the temperature goes up very quickly and the child convulses (see section on Convulsions).

Of course, when your child has a fever you will watch closely for signs of illness, and question him/her about any complaints s/he may have. If your child has a fever and acts unusually sleepy or irritable, or has specific complaints, you will want to take a health history, asking such questions as are found in Chapter 2.

*Physical signs.* The first and most important objective assessment of fever is to measure the child's temperature. Sometimes, in deciding to give some specific remedy to a child, it is very helpful to know whether there has been any fever, and if so, how high that fever has been and what pattern it has taken over the cycle of the day. Even experienced mothers (and doctors) are unable to judge reliably the amount of fever by the time-honored method of feeling the child's forehead with the back of the hand or with the cheek. While there is no need to measure temperature compulsively every four hours, do be thoughtful about getting a measurement when you think there is a change at the beginning or end of an illness. Remember to take the temperature before you give aspirin or an aspirin substitute, or four hours after you have given fever medicine, when its effects have worn off.

After measuring the temperature, and if your child has complaints or is acting ill, you will want to examine him/her for indications of specific illness. No matter what the complaints it is always good to check the respiratory system (including the ears, nose, throat, and the lungs), the belly, the skin, and the nervous system, including a check for a stiff neck. Even if your child has no complaints and seems to feel well, you should do this kind of examination if s/he has had fever for as long as 48 hours.

You will want to get professional consultation if your feverish child has any of the following problems:

- A stiff neck.
- Excessive sleepiness, difficult to arouse.
- A convulsion or excessive jitteryness that does not go away when the temperature is brought down by aspirin or aspirin substitute.
- A red or swollen joint.
- Severe pain anywhere, even if it goes away with aspirin; if the pain reappears after the effect of the aspirin wears off in four hours, its cause should be ascertained.
- Dehydration, shown by a dry mouth, infrequent voiding of urine, and a doughy feel to the skin.
- Any indication of bleeding into or under the skin — many unexplained black-and-blue marks or fine points of bleeding, like a fine, flat red rash, just under the surface of the skin, called petechiae.
- Breathing difficulty — noisy breathing in or out, or breathing that is slower than usual or faster than usual.
- A high fever (above 39.2°C/102.6°F by rectum or

38.7°C/101.6°F by mouth) of 48 hours' duration, or a low-grade fever (above 38.1°C/100.6°F by rectum or 37.6°C/99.6°F by mouth) of 4 days' duration, for which you can find no explanation by thinking about what illnesses the child has been exposed to, what complaints s/he has, and what you find when you examine him/her.

A fever in an infant less than 4 months old should always be checked by a professional. Small babies do not react to infections and other kinds of illnesses in the same fashion as older children, and they can become very ill in a very short time. Fortunately, they also recover very quickly.

*Other things you should know.* There is some suggestion from research that having a fever offers the body an advantage in fighting against infections. We should think of reasons for trying to reduce fever. If a child seems to be very uncomfortable or can't sleep, it makes sense to try to reduce the fever and then see if the child seems to feel more comfortable (there might be reasons for the distress other than the fever). If the child is very jittery, or very sleepy, try to bring down the fever. If the jitteryness or sleepiness goes away, they are probably, in this instance, a direct effect of the fever. If the child has had seizures before with a fever, you will want to try to keep the temperature below the level at which the seizure occurred on the previous occasion.

Otherwise, there is little reason to try vigorously to bring down fever, remembering that it might be helpful to the child in the healing process. Consider instead how to make the child as comfortable as possible to help the body heal itself.

Our bodies deal with fever by getting rid of the excess heat in a variety of ways:

- More rapid breathing carries heat from the lungs.
- Heat is given off from the surface of the skin, especially if there is a slight air current.
- If the surface of the skin is wet (as with sweating), more heat is carried away.

If cooling is too rapid, our bodies *increase* body temperature by shivering. A chill, therefore, often means that body temperature is going up. Understanding these natural bodily reactions to fever helps us to plan treatments for a child with a fever.

Most high fevers of sudden onset are due to short-term infections, such as infections of the throat, the ears, the upper breathing passages, the lungs, the stomach and gut, and the urinary system. Fevers can also be a sign of dehydration, over-exertion, prolonged exposure to hot sun, lack of sufficient salt replacement for excessive sweating, reactions to drugs, malignant tumors, diseases of the connective tissue like ar-thritis, and other rare kinds of illness. Not all fevers are ex-plained. Often a child develops a fever and has no specific signs of illness — other than, perhaps, crankiness, a decreased appetite, and an apparent need for extra sleep. The fever soon goes away, leaving no clear-cut explanation for its cause. Doc-tors often say that teething does not cause fever, because no one knows how (by what mechanism) that might happen. Nonetheless, babies who are cutting teeth (or are showing signs that teeth are working their way through gums) sometimes have brief fevers with no other cause being evident.

*Remedies.* The first and most important remedies for fever are those that support the child's own natural bodily processes.

- Don't dress the child warmly. Use light clothing, and per-haps a light sheet for comfort, to allow a child the chance to get rid of body heat by the circulation of room air.
- If it makes the child feel good, turn on a fan. A cool-mist vaporizer (which you will want to use for respiratory in-fections) will also produce a movement of cool air.
- Wiping the child's skin with a cool (not cold) damp cloth — especially with something good-smelling in the water — will also help rid the body of heat.
- Sitting the child in a tub full of room-temperature (not cold) water with some toys to play with will also bring the temperature down.

In all of the above remedies, the most important signal is the child's comfort. If what you are doing feels good, it is probably the right thing to do. Specifically, do not sponge the child with ice water — it is very uncomfortable. Do not sponge the child with alcohol — the chilling effect is too sudden and

too great, and little children have even become somewhat in-
toxicated by alcohol fumes! If the drop in body temperature is
fast enough, the brain will react and signal the child's body to
shiver. Shivering and teeth-chattering are indications that the
body is trying to warm itself, and your efforts are getting
nowhere.

Offer the child lots of extra liquids to drink. Follow the
child's lead for preferred drinks — his/her body probably
knows what is needed. Follow the child's lead also about the
temperature of the drink. If the child has a sore mouth or sore
throat, or is nauseated, an iced drink will probably taste best.
On the other hand, cold drinks may increase the body's temperature because the liquid needs to be warmed by the body
to its own temperature. The child may prefer a drink at room
temperature or body temperature. (None of this needs to be
measured precisely.) Remember that warm drinks — especially
those with a spicey substance added, such as cayenne pepper
or ginger — tend to make the body sweat and increase cooling
in that way. A cool-mist vaporizer helps keep the body hy-
drated by making the air more humid, but is no substitute for
the extra drinking that is needed to make up for sweating and
for the extra water needed by the body for ordinary metabolic
processes.

These remedies may suffice to make the child comfortable
and bring down a high temperature. There are, in addition,
two drugs that bring down fever; both seem to work on the
central nervous system. The first is aspirin. Some authorities
believe that aspirin is the most effective fever-reducing drug.
It is not made in a liquid form, but aspirin tablets can be
chewed (child-dose aspirin tablets are made with flavoring) or
crushed and mixed with applesauce, honey, or granulated
sugar. The dose of aspirin for a child is 10–15 mgm/K, or
100–150 mgm/22 pounds, given every 4 hours. Plain aspirin
tablets (or aspirin suppositories) can also be given by rectum,
for a child who is vomiting or who is too cranky to cooperate
in swallowing the drug. Aspirin should not be given more than
4 times in 24 hours, if you are giving aspirin for more than
one 24-hour period.

Some children cannot take aspirin. Some are allergic to the drug — an allergy that often runs in families. Some cannot take the drug because they have a specific metabolic individuality, called G6PD deficiency (see p. 310) Sometimes people with ulcers or bleeding tendencies are advised not to take aspirin. In these cases, another drug called acetoaminophen can be taken. This drug can be prepared in liquid form and is therefore easier to give to a child, but it may not be as effective in reducing fever as aspirin is. The dose of acetoaminophen for a child is 60 mgm for a child of less than one year of age, 90 mgm between the first and third birthday, 120 mgm between the third and sixth birthday, and 240 mgm after the sixth birthday.

Both of these drugs — like all drugs — have side effects. It is not clear that acetoaminophen has fewer or less serious side effects than aspirin; certainly it is a newer drug than aspirin and has not been studied as carefully. For those who cannot take aspirin, acetoaminophen is the appropriate drug. However, one should not give *any* drug without good reason.

Always with a fever of any significant height or duration you will want to review the need for other remedies, based on what you know about the child's recent activities and your physical examination of the child.


## Foreign Bodies in Holes

Children love to stick things into things. Sometimes they stick things into parts of themselves, and the objects become trapped. The most common places for troublesome foreign bodies are the windpipe, the nose, the ears, and the vagina.

*Personal symptoms.* It is helpful to know what small objects your child likes to play with, and what body parts hold fascination for him/her. Many mothers are entirely surprised to learn that a child has stuck some foreign object into his/her body.

Foreign bodies in the windpipe are the most likely to be dangerous. If a bean or bead gets stuck centrally, it can stop breathing. This is an emergency, to which one responds with the old and familiar technique of turning the child over one's knee and slapping the child's back between the shoulder blades. The object will usually be dislodged with one or two sharp slaps.

A small object can also get stuck in one side or the other of the windpipe after it branches. In this case it will cause a frequent nonproductive cough, and sometimes a whistley, wheezy sound to the breathing.

Foreign bodies in other holes cause discomfort, sometimes, and often a pussy, smelly discharge; this is true for the ear, the nose, and the vagina.

*Physical signs.* A foreign body in the ear can be seen with an otoscope. The same instrument can also be used to look into the nose.

A foreign body on one side of the large breathing tubes can be guessed at if the breathing on the two sides sounds different when you listen with a stethoscope. You must always pay attention to this comparison when a child has a short, frequent, nonproductive cough. The side without the foreign body will sound normal. The side with the foreign body may have a sound like wheezing (in or out), or may have no breath sounds at all if the object completely obstructs the breathing tube.

A foreign body in the vagina can be felt by using a rubber glove or a rubber finger cover, applying a liberal amount of petroleum jelly, and inserting a finger into the child's rectum. To do this you push gently against her anus, instructing her to breath with a shallow pant like a puppy. This will distract her and relax her abdominal muscles; sometimes she will also relax the ring of muscles around her anus. If you push steadily against her anus your finger will slip in. When it slips in, reassure your child that it will not hurt her for your finger to be there, but only feel as if she has to make a bowel movement.

The vagina lies just in front of the rectum; as the child lies on her back the vagina lies just above where your finger is. Pushing upward, run your finger along the length of the vagina; any small object feels like a lump against your finger.

This is one of those examinations we would all rather not

do since it is somewhat uncomfortable for the child. You will have to decide whether you, who know her well and can reassure her, would rather do this examination, or whether you would rather have it done by a stranger. If she is preadolescent and has a copious and smelly discharge that is clearly coming from her vagina, this examination will need to be done.

*Remedies.* Some foreign bodies of the nose and the ear can be removed at home. It takes a long tweezers and a steady hand to do so. Food objects like beans and peanuts usually swell if they have remained in place for long, and, as a consequence, become very firmly lodged. If the object cannot be easily removed you should ask for professional help. Professionals have special implements and special techniques for removing such objects that do not hurt the child.

Foreign bodies in the respiratory tract must be located by X-ray. They can usually be removed by a procedure called bronchoscopy. This involves inserting a long hollow pipe, with a light on the end, down into the breathing tube, and using a long pincerlike implement to reach down into the pipe and grasp the object. This is done under general anesthesia, in most cases.

Foreign bodies in the vagina are removed through a similar but much shorter tube. They can usually be removed without anesthesia; if the child is upset by the procedure she can be lightly sedated by drugs.

Of all of these accidents, the most serious in its consequences is that of a foreign body in the breathing tubes. To prevent all such accidents would require a kind of vigilance that might be of psychological detriment to a child. But it is well to be aware of the bits and pieces that your infant and toddler finds and puts into his/her mouth. Children who are coughing from respiratory infections are especially likely to inhale some foreign object put casually into the mouth.

## Headache

A headache may be a localized or overall pain in any part of the head; it can be steady or throbbing, of short duration or lasting for hours or even days, and may be caused by a wide variety of precipitating events.

*Personal symptoms.* Small children rarely complain of headache. This may be because they are not prone to the happenings that cause headache in adults, because they experience pain differently than adults do, or because they have difficulty reporting the sensations of headache. As children grow toward adolescence they are increasingly likely to complain of headache. Television advertising for headache remedies seems sometimes to be the direct precipitant of a complaint of headache in a bored child!

The sinus spaces in the face continue to develop throughout childhood; children rarely have sinus trouble as adults do. But nasal congestion from allergy does sometimes seem to be a cause of headache in children; the ache is described as around the eyes and the nose.

Eye strain, in a child who needs glasses, is perhaps the most easily diagnosed and treated cause of headache in children. This headache is described as around the eyes and forehead, on both sides, and comes on after a period of using the eyes for close work. A child with eye strain may have recurrent headaches after school that clear by the time s/he has walked home.

Some of us cannot maintain adequate blood sugar levels without frequent small meals of protein. The condition of hypoglycemia (low blood sugar) can cause headache and a faint feeling. In school children, whose mealtimes are determined by school rules, this kind of generalized whole-head ache will appear after an interval of not eating.

An ache at the back of the head, sometimes especially noticeable on arising from sleep, is sometimes seen with high blood pressure. High blood pressure is relatively rare in children and is usually a part of some specific disease, such as a kidney disease. Any child who complains of chronic headache should have his/her blood pressure measured.

Children have migraine headaches. Those who do are likely to have a family history of migraine or of allergies. Migraine headaches are often one-sided and usually recur at regular intervals in a repetitive pattern.

A headache can be an early manifestation of brain disease of a variety of sorts. Your observation of the child's day-to-day capabilities, and a professional's careful assessment of the child's neurological status (including examination of the eyes with an ophthalmoscope) are both necessary to consider the possibility of this diagnosis. More complex tests, some performed only in hospitals, may be needed to investigate brain anatomy and function if this diagnosis seems a likelihood.

Most headaches in children, like those in adults, are the result of fatigue, worry, and tension. A headache is one of the body's most common ways of saying, "Slow down, find some peace and quiet, retreat from vigorous striving; you need rest and a chance to think about yourself and your world."

*Physical signs.* A child with frequent headaches that cannot be managed by home remedies, and that cause the child to miss school or play to an excessive degree, should be examined by a professional. In home examination, you will want to:

- check the blood pressure
- examine the urine
- observe gait, balance, and speech carefully for recent changes
- tap about the nose and above the eyes to search for tenderness in the sinus areas.

Headaches with fever are common, and are usually explained by the process that has caused the fever.

*Remedies.* Headaches caused by eyestrain, sinus congestion, and high blood pressure require professional assistance in their remedies. Migraine headaches can be relieved or warded off by combinations of drug treatment, under the supervision of a professional.

Simple headaches from fatigue, worry, and tension can be treated at home. See Chapter 4, section on Aspirin, for a discussion of remedies for these types of headaches.

## Head Trauma

Head trauma is any blow or injury to the head.

*Personal symptoms.* Children fall or stumble so frequently that few get through their early years without a worrisome

blow to the head. Toddlers who move more quickly and im-
pulsively than their neuromotor development can control, and
who fall repeatedly, usually fall in the same way each time. I
have seen youngsters with foreheads "calloused" from falling.
Their falls cause swelling and a breakage of tissue under the
skin, and the growth of connective tissue as part of the healing
process. When this sequence of events is repeated many times
there can develop a firm pad of tissue just under the skin, as
if for protection against repeated bumps.

The most helpful thing to know about a blow to the head
is how it happened and how the child acted immediately after.
If you did not see the accident you will want to question
closely anyone who was with the child at the time that it
happened. It is important to know what part of the head was
hit, and what it was hit with. Did the child cry immediately,
indicating that there was no period of unconsciousness? Did
the child lie very still for a few moments, suggesting that s/he
was "out"? Was the skin broken? Was there any bleeding? Did
the child get up spontaneously or did someone pick the child
up? Was there any indication at any time that the child could
not see well? Did both arms and both legs move in a normal
fashion? In the interval after the accident, was there any change
in the child's normal behavior? How were balance and coordination? Was there vomiting? Did the child seem unusually
irritable?

It is important not to forget to ask whether the child seems
to have been injured anywhere else other than on the head.

*Physical signs.* Examination of a child with a head injury
begins with the place of injury. Is there a laceration? If there
is a cut deep enough that the edges fall apart it should be
sutured so that the wound does not get infected. (There will
also be less scar with suturing, but most of us don't care much
about scars on the scalp.) Lacerations of the scalp can bleed
excessively; the bleeding can be stopped by the firm application of a clean cloth.

There are three kinds of head injury that should be
checked by a professional. One is an injury to the side of the
head, around and above the ears. A skull fracture in this area

can tear an artery that lies just under the bone, causing quick and massive bleeding. This is an injury that is potentially life-threatening and sometimes needs emergency surgery.

Another kind of injury that needs to be checked is one that results in a soft, boggy swelling such that you cannot feel with your fingers whether the underlying bone is intact. In this case it is often a good idea to get an X-ray to be sure that there is not a sliver of bone pressing on the brain underneath.

Other kinds of head injury are not likely to be dangerous unless the child's response to the injury suggests that some damage has been done. Any suggestion of a disturbance of eyesight, a markedly altered capacity for coordination and balance, vomiting more than once, unusual sleepiness (coma or an inability to be aroused) either immediately after the accident or at any time in the next 24 hours, and prolonged crying and irritability require examination and assessment by a professional.

Trouble for a child who has had a head injury will in most cases appear within 24 hours. You should allow the child to follow his/her regular routine as s/he wishes (although it would be well that the child did not play so excitedly that s/he might fall and hit the head again). Naps and meals can proceed as usual, according to the child's willingness.

You should check the child every 3 hours for the next 24 hours, to be sure that no signs of brain injury have appeared. Wake the child from sleeping to do this. Look at the eyes, to be sure that they move together and that the pupils are the same size. Chat with the child about things in the room to be sure that s/he can see as well as usual. Have the child walk, to check balance and coordination, and be sure s/he can move all four limbs. Talk with the child to be sure that the child is his/her usual sensible self. If you find a change in condition, consult a professional.

The most frequently seen long-term aftereffect of a head injury occurs because of slow bleeding under the dura, the tough membrane that covers the brain. In a baby whose skull bones are not grown together this will result in increased head size; in an older child (in whom this condition is more unusual) there is no change in head size but an increase in pressure on the brain by the space-occupying fluid. In this condition (called a subdural hematoma) the child will show increasingly disturbed behavior: excessive sleepiness or irritability, vomiting, poor feeding, and restless sleeping. This condition is very rare, but mothers are most likely to notice the signs of its presence. It can and should be treated.

*Remedies.* The major remedy for head injuries is to try to minimize their occurrence. Child safety is too big and important a topic to be dealt with thoroughly here, but needs to be thought about by mothers every day. A reminder for those who seat young babies in slant-angled infant seats: those seats must be very firmly anchored, especially if the seat is placed on a table or counter top, for it is very easy for the baby to wiggle and fall to the floor, the seat landing on top of him/her.

A child who has had a head injury and seems otherwise all right should have an aspirin if s/he complains (reasonably so) of a headache. Never give codeine or any stronger pain medicine to a child who has had a head injury.

A scalp laceration that does not have gaping edges can be washed and covered with a sterile dressing. Wash the wound well with Betadyne or pHisohex soap after trimming the hair around the wound with a razor or small scissors. Cover it with a small piece of nonadherent dressing and then a pad of gauze. Fix the dressing in place by tying small strands of hair over the dressing (tape will not stick to hair). Check the wound daily and replace the dressing until the surface of the wound is crusted and dry. Your child needs a tetanus booster only if s/he has not had one within the last two months, if s/he is less than 5 years old, or within the last ten years, if s/he is older than 5 years.

## Inflammatory Rashes

Rashes that are primarily inflammatory respond to steroid drugs.

Steroid drugs are synthetic substances that have the properties of the hormones manufactured by human adrenal glands; these substances combat inflammation.

*Personal symptoms.* There are a variety of nonspecific rashes that are primarily inflammatory. They are usually dry and often itchy; they may be red or may have little color change from normal skin.

Many steroid-responsive rashes have an allergic basis. With careful thought you may be able to identify the offending substance. Rashes that appear in only one area of the body are usually the result of contact with an allergenic substance. Rashes that are generalized, or that appear in the inner surfaces of the elbows, are likely to result from eating an allergenic food or breathing in an allergenic substance in the air. Allergic rashes are often mysterious, and one may discover the cause-and-effect linkage only after several repeated episodes.

Eczema, a generalized allergic rash appearing on the inner surfaces of the elbows and cheeks, as well as elsewhere on the body, can be worsened by emotional stress and by the dryness of winter air in houses.

*Physical signs.* Steroids only deal with inflammation and can actually worsen an infection. Rashes resulting from viral infection usually are accompanied by other symptoms: fever, cough, sore throat, and so on.

Rashes with local bacteria or fungal infection are usually cracked and oozing or crusted; if the infection is bacterial the oozing material will appear clear and yellowish or pussy.

*Remedies.* Even with all the cautions about ruling out rashes due to infection, there remain many, many rashes — usually never completely explained — that respond to treatment with steroid drugs.

Steroids taken by mouth have known hazardous side effects. Oral administration of steroids for children should be reserved for very serious illness in which the risk of harm is less than the potentially harmful outcome of the disease itself.

Steroid salves, however, are very useful in skin care for children. A dry, itchy, inflammatory condition that persists for a week or ten days will often disappear dramatically after a few applications of a steroid salve. Many rashes, of course, need no specific treatment.

The least expensive preparation is hydrocortisone cream, 1%. It should be applied thinly, three or four times a day. It is only available by prescription.

## Insect Bites

Insect bites usually cause some variety of a typical lesion called a wheal-and-flare: there is a central raised area that is sometimes pale, and an irregular red halo surrounding the central area.

*Personal symptoms.* Different people react differently to insect bites; some are very bothered in one way or another, and some are bothered almost not at all. These are some of the insects that most commonly bite children:

- Mosquitos are summer insects in temperate climates. They usually cause small to moderate wheal-and-flare bumps.
- Black flies are early summer insects. They usually hurt when they bite, and can cause fairly large bumps.
- "No-see-ums" (which have a variety of local names) are so tiny that they are often not seen; they can come through window screens. They are not very common in cities. Their bites usually cause very small bumps.
- Fleas travel on cats, dogs, and other furry household pets. They are most likely to be bothersome in mid to late fall, and go away after the first freeze. One flea can get inside a sock, or a pajama top, and make several bites in a small area so that the skin looks as if it has a localized rash. Putting flea collars on the pets may help keep the flea population down, but it is important *not* to keep the pets outside. The fleas in the house (in the rugs, on the furniture) are better on the pets than on the people. Flea bites are usually small, round, and red.
- Spiders appear at different times of the year in different localities. Tiny household spiders can get into a child's bed and cause several bites in one night. Spider bites are very small but can cause intense itch.

- Bees, hornets, and wasps are the insects whose bites are most likely to cause a severe allergic reaction, called an anaphylactic reaction, resulting in breathing difficulty and a fall in blood pressure. This is a medical emergency. An anaphylactic reaction rarely occurs the first time a child is bitten, but if the first bite results in a very large wheal-and-flare, or causes generalized hives, you should be watchful about a second bite. All of these insects give a bite that is painful immediately.

The above are the most common insects to plague babies and children. There are rare poisonous insects that give bites with serious consequences. There are also special local insects. One needs to know what insects are common locally, and at what time of year they appear.

Deciding exactly what insect caused a bite is usually difficult and uncertain unless you saw the insect make the bite. Usually we make a guess based on experience. Except when there is a danger of an anaphylactic reaction, it is usually not necessary to know what made the bite in order to treat the child's distress. But it is helpful in preventing later bites to try to determine what the insect was, in order to get rid of the insect or protect the child.

Bites can be painful immediately at the time of the bite. They can also cause, for a variable period of time, a sensation of warmth and/or itching.

*Physical signs.* Insect bites can vary from one gigantic wheal-and-flare (covering a whole upper arm, or most of the back) to tiny raised red bumps. They can disappear in a matter of minutes, or remain visible for days. If they are itchy and the child scratches, all evidence of the bite can disappear under scratch marks and open oozing sores. Bites around the eyes and the ears can cause swelling that is disfiguring.

*Other things you should know.* Small babies are not likely to be bothered by itch from insect bites because the nerves of the skin that carry the sensation of itch (which is a kind of mild pain) are relatively immature and inefficient. But when there are biting insects around, an unprotected baby can become physically ill from a multitude of bites. The baby may simply sleep through the attack of the insects. If you or older children are being bitten, do protect the baby with netting.

Remember that some biting insects carry serious disease — mosquitos, fleas, and ticks can carry such disease. This information, of course, is specific to particular localities.

If your family has a history of anaphylactic reaction to insect bites, a child may not be so afflicted but is certainly more at risk than other children. If these reactions have occurred in close family members, or have been very severe, you will want always to have an anaphylaxis kit (see below) at hand.

*Remedies.* The simplest preventive remedy is thiamine, vitamin $B_1$, taken by mouth. The dose for a two-year-old is 50 mgm each day; for an eight-year-old, 100 mgm; and for an adult, 200 mgm each day. It is suspected that this vitamin changes the skin or body secretions so that one no longer tastes or smells good to insects. Bothersome side effects have not been reported for this remedy, but as with all special-purpose substances one should take thiamine tablets only for that period of time when the risk of severe insect bites is very troublesome.

Be very restrained in applying insect repellents to small children, and do not use them at all for small babies. All contain chemicals that are potentially hazardous, especially to little people. Many contain chemicals that can burn eyes, noses, and mouths, and small children will put their hands in all of these places.

Remedies for the immediate pain of insect bites are the following:

- An ice cube held to the bite.
- If you see a stinger — a fine, dark-colored thread — in the center of the bite, it can be removed with tweezers.
- A poultice of cornstarch and water, or baking soda and water.
- A poultice of water mixed with meat tenderizer, containing the enzyme papain.
  Remedies for the itch of insect bites are:
- Aspirin.

- A compress of very warm water — as warm as can be tolerated, but not so warm as to burn the skin.
- Compresses or baths with one of the following: baking soda, cornstarch, or colloidal oatmeal (regular oatmeal is equally soothing but clogs up the drains).
- Calamine lotion.
- Something distracting to do.
- If the child scratches at bites in his/her sleep, put socks over the hands or pin over the hands of her pajamas. Scratching can cause open sores and even a superficial infection, impetigo.

There is also an itch medicine that can be taken by mouth, called Benadryl. This is an antihistamine and acts on the central nervous system, which seems to be a strong remedy for a symptom that is ordinarily rather mild and responsive to more simple treatment.

For some parents, the major problem with insect bites is cosmetic. Children with many bites can look spotty and swollen. If the child is not bothered, there is little reason to treat the disfigurement.

Unless there is a true anaphylactic reaction, there is no reason to treat insect bites with steroid drugs. Steroids given orally take many hours to have an effect, and by then the bites are likely to cause little or no trouble. Steroids also have known and predictable side effects that interfere with the body's metabolism and ability to deal with stress.

Anaphylaxis is a rare but serious consequence of an insect bite. The symptoms of difficult breathing and shock (from a sudden fall in blood pressure) appear almost immediately, certainly within the first hour after the bite. If your child or your child's family history has so strong a tendency to allergy that there seems to be a possibility of anaphylaxis, you should carry a special kit to treat this reaction. The kit can be made up with professional help, or it can be bought already made up. You should get careful instruction in the use of the kit from a doctor, nurse, or other medical professional trained in emergency medicine. As with all medical and surgical emergencies that are life-threatening, home treatment in this case is only a temporary (although a potentially life-saving) remedy. You should begin immediately to make arrangements — by car, police vehicle, or ambulance — to get the child to an emergency room.

## Lead Poisoning

Lead poisoning is said to exist when the amount of lead circulating in the child's blood exceeds some arbitrary level, usually set at 40 micrograms percent.

*Personal symptoms.* Lead does not normally occur in the human body. It serves no use. Lead is a cellular poison, with a special propensity for damaging the cells of the central nervous system. Because the nervous system and brain of the young are growing and developing rapidly, a child is especially susceptible to damage from lead poisoning.

The most important clue to lead poisoning is your suspicion that the child might be exposed to lead. If you are suspicious, it is relatively easy to have your child's blood tested for lead.

There are many sources of lead in our modern environment, including cigarette smoke (tobacco is often treated with a lead-containing chemical in the fields). The two most important sources of lead for children are chipping and falling paint, and the fumes from vehicles that burn lead-containing gasoline. One can take in lead by inhaling it or by eating it.

Most old houses have lead-containing paint on the walls, inside and out. If that paint is chipped and falling, the child may pick up bits to eat, lay a doughnut down on the paint chips of a window sill, or eat paint dust that falls into food in the kitchen. Some children gnaw or lick at painted windowsills and crib bars.

The lead level in the air in places where there are many moving cars and trucks can be quite high. Children who live or play in areas where there is a lot of traffic are also at risk of lead poisoning.

Children with levels of lead in their bodies that are high enough to be considered dangerous may not show any symptoms. In any case, the symptoms of mild lead poisoning (at a level that damages cells but does not make the child severely ill) are very nonspecific: they include irritability, hyperactivity, listlessness, poor appetite, and a diminished capacity to learn.

*Physical signs.* With one exception, there is no examination of the child that you can do at home that will help you learn whether or not your child is poisoned with lead. That exception is the fine dark bluish line that can be seen at the point where the gums lie up against the teeth. This "lead line" usually appears only after children have been exposed to lead for a long time.

Most states and local governments now have lead-detection and deleading programs for houses; as part of these programs children can be tested for lead poisoning. Ask your doctor. Unfortunately, many doctors still believe that lead poisoning is only a problem of poor children, and give false reassurance to mothers who are not poor. If your doctor does not do lead testing and cannot refer you to a place that does, call your state or local department or board of health.

*Remedies.* The most important remedy for lead poisoning is prevention. Houses and apartments can be deleaded for about $100 per room. Since the lead of paint soaks into plaster and wood it is usually more practical to cover walls that have been painted with lead, and to remove and replace old woodwork. Before deleading, an inspection should be done of the house to determine which painted or plastered areas have lead. The inspection, advice on deleading, and sometimes part of the actual work of deleading may be done by your local lead program. In rented apartments and houses it is the landlord's responsibility to delead; enforcement of this law has been very difficult, for obvious reasons.

Children who are poisoned with lead can be treated with drugs that remove some of the lead from the child's body. There are different treatments for children who are very ill with lead poisoning (for instance, with convulsions or coma) and for children who do not show specific signs of illness but are known to have dangerously high levels of lead in their blood.

Lead in the body damages cells when it circulates in the blood. It is also stored in many organs, notably in the bones. Just as with the molecules of calcium in the bones, the molecules of lead move in and out of their storage sites in bone. This means that more cellular damage can occur whenever a large amount of lead recirculates in the blood. The lead washes out of and is later redeposited in bone. Because of this storage-and-release phenomenon, any treatment to remove lead from a child's body must be continued for some time.

Lead poisoning is a serious problem for children. The most important preventive measures involve removing the lead from the environment. This is an effort that requires more than the energies of individual parents to be successful. It requires organized community effort, at the local, state, and national level.

## Leukemia

Leukemia is a malignant change of the tissues that form blood; it is serious, treatable, but sometimes fatal.

*Personal symptoms.* Leukemia is not treatable only by home-care skills, although much of the treatment for leukemia is done at home. It is included here primarily because it is an illness that mothers often worry about; its onset is often vague and insidious and its initial symptoms nonspecific.

Among the first symptoms of leukemia are that familiar trio, crankiness, poor appetite, and easy fatigue. Obviously, these are simply signals that a child is not feeling well; one must wait and see what illness develops from these initial clues. Because leukemia results in changes in the composition of the blood, the most characteristic symptoms of leukemia reflect the functions of blood. There is a change in the blood's ability to clot; as a consequence, there is easy bruising and prolonged bleeding from minor cuts and abrasions. There is a malfunction of the cells that protect against infection; therefore there is difficulty in warding off and overcoming ordinary childhood infections. There is also a decrease in the red blood cells that carry hemoglobin, so that there is anemia with pallor and easy fatigue.

*Physical signs.* The initial physical signs of leukemia —
in addition to those that reflect the changes in blood function
described above — are the enlargement of the organs that form
blood, including lymph nodes everywhere in the body and
the liver and spleen. However, no illness events and no physical signs are absolutely characteristic of leukemia. The diagnosis is made by examining the blood-forming tissue itself.
Examination of the blood-forming tissue is done by aspirating
a bit of bone marrow and looking at it under the microscope.
This is a minor surgical procedure and is done in a hospital or
clinic.

*Remedies.* Leukemia is now treated with a variety of very
potent drugs, most of which have harmful as well as beneficial
effects. The drugs (and other treatments) are given in a pro-
gramed succession, in an effort to maximize the beneficial
effects and to minimize the harmful effects. These are indeed
heroic treatments. Children with leukemia now have a reasonable prognosis for months or years of near-normal life, although at the time of initial diagnosis it is still difficult to say
what the course will be for the individual child.

## Mononucleosis

Mononucleosis is a disease of relatively low contagiousness,
caused by a virus, that usually begins with acute symptoms
and runs a slow course to complete recovery.

*Personal symptoms.* Although mononucleosis is ordinarily a disease of adolescents and young adults, it is also experienced by young children. One rarely knows the source of
contagion. Initial symptoms may be sleepiness, irritability, a
drop in appetite, a fever, and often a sore throat. In its beginning stages the illness often appears to be like a strep throat.

As the disease develops, there may be a variety of additional symptoms. Belly ache and vomiting, a stiff neck, cough,
and headache are common. In other children there may be few
specific symptoms, the disease expressing itself primarily as a
prolonged fatigability and crankiness.

*Physical signs.* The nodes in the neck are often enlarged;

nodes in the armpits and groin are also likely to be larger than usual, and sometimes tender. The throat may be reddened and may have some white exudate, looking like the so-called typical picture of a strep throat. There may be a skin rash that looks like many other rashes of viral disease — fine, red, and slightly raised. Although a stiff neck may be only the consequence of enlarged lymph nodes, stiff neck and headache suggest some degree of meningoencephalitis. Enlargement and dysfunction of the liver and the spleen sometimes occur. You may be able to feel the outlines of these organs when you examine the belly, or you may only elicit some tenderness as you feel. Significant dysfunction of the liver may be expressed by jaundice, a yellow color to the skin and the whites of the eyes; this is best seen in daylight rather than in artificial light.

A throat culture should be done if you suspect the possibility of a strep throat. Professional consultation should be sought if there is persistent high fever, a marked headache, a stiff neck that does not flex forward with ease, jaundice, or markedly enlarged or tender liver or spleen.

A definite diagnosis of mononucleosis is given by the results of laboratory tests. The cell count of the blood shows an increase and predominance of lymph cells (one kind of white cell) with an abnormal form to many of those lymph cells. There is a specific antibody test for mononucleosis that usually does not confirm the presence of the disease until a week to ten days after the onset of symptoms. Therefore if the initial throat culture shows that the sore throat, fever, and swollen glands are not due to a strep infection, consultation with a professional should wait for a week to ten days in the absence of the other signs and symptoms, indicated above.

One does not diagnose mononucleosis in order to offer a remedy, because there is no specific treatment for mononucleosis. The reason for trying to pin down the diagnosis is to know what to expect in terms of convalescence, and to know that the child will not get that disease again.

Convalescence from mononucleosis often lasts as long as six months for an adolescent, but generally runs a shorter course in a younger child. That lengthy recovery period does not necessarily involve absence from school or an inability to carry on regular activities. It does, however, mean that the child will complain of easy fatigue, seem more irritable or edgy than usual, and have a tendency to come down with other minor infections.

*Remedies.* Treatment for mononucleosis is entirely symptomatic and supportive. Rest, when the child indicates, and a nourishing and supportive diet are the primary needs of the convalescent child. S/he may need help in arranging to keep up with schoolwork. Reassurance that the child will, in time, regain accustomed levels of energy and enthusiasm is important. Patience with any irritability, and reasonable expectations for accommodation of other household members will help the child understand him/herself as s/he slowly returns to the usual healthy state.

## Mumps

Mumps is an infection caused by a virus that has a special affinity for glandular and nervous tissue. Most cases of mumps occur in preadolescent children. As with most of the common diseases of childhood, the disease is usually more distressful when it is experienced after adolescence.

*Personal symptoms.* In the early phase of the disease, there may be crankiness, fever, the complaint of a sore neck or jaw, and headache. Mumps is relatively noncontagious so that not all children who are exposed to another child ill with mumps will themselves come down with the disease. As always, however, when your child begins to show signs of illness you will want to find out whether s/he may have been exposed to some particular illness. The incubation period (time from exposure until the appearance of the first symptoms) for mumps is two to three weeks.

As the disease develops, there is a characteristic swelling of the salivary gland in front of the ear. Although in some cases of mumps these glands are not affected, it is very difficult to be sure that the child has mumps if this characteristic sign is not present. The child will complain of pain in front of the ear or over the angle of the jaw. Drinking acidic liquids like orange juice causes a sudden spurt of secretion of saliva and may cause pain in the salivary duct (at the inside of the cheek) affected by the infection. Since the mumps virus also has some affinity for other glands, there may be complaints of pain under the jaw (where there are other salivary glands), in the center of the neck (the thyroid gland), in the upper belly (the pancreas), the lower belly (the ovaries), the scrotum (the testes), or the upper eyelids (the lacrimal glands). Involvement of glands other than the salivary glands is less common in young children than in adolescents. The affinity of the virus for nervous tissue may cause muscular aches and severe headache. When there is severe headache it is usually assumed that the virus has caused a meningoencephalitis, an inflammation of the covering of the brain (the meninges) and of the brain tissue itself. Most virus infections are bloodstream infections and can potentially invade any organ of the body. The occurrence of headache in any viral infection suggests some degree, however mild, of meningoencephalitis. Meningoencephalitis is therefore a fairly common infection, and usually has no aftereffects.

*Physical signs.* Even before there is visible swelling of the parotid glands there may be tenderness in front of the ear. The gland extends in front of the ear down along the jaw and often over the angle of the jaw into the neck. Lymph nodes, on the other hand, do not usually extend up over the angle of the jaw into the area of the cheek. Swollen lymph nodes in the side of the neck should be easily distinguished from the parotid swelling of mumps.

Once the parotid swelling of mumps is well developed, the child's appearance is quite characteristic. There is a chipmunklike swelling of the cheek; the earlobe is pushed upward and outward.

The opening of the duct from the affected parotid gland is inside the cheek opposite the molars; you may be able to see it as a small red spot. The child usually has fever while the swelling is developing, after which the fever goes down close to normal. Only when the swelling has subsided does the temperature return to normal. If, as is often the case, the involvement of various glands occurs in a sequence, the temperature may be rather high, then go down close to normal, then be high again, then lower, then high again, and so on.

Inflammation of the ovaries and testicles, and the inflammation of meningoencephalitis, usually occurs after both parotid glands have been affected. These are the most commonly recognized complications of simple mumps. Any gland affected by the mumps virus will be swollen and tender.

*Other things you should know.* In about one-quarter of cases only one parotid gland is affected. Inflammation of the ovaries and the testes is usually confined to only one side. Sterility almost never results from this infection.

There are other much more rare complications of mumps. Among these are arthritis, a fall in the number of circulating platelets (which are necessary for the clotting of blood), and deafness.

The child should be considered contagious until all swelling, tenderness, and pain have disappeared, and the temperature has returned to normal.

*Remedies.* There is no specific treatment for mumps. One makes the child as comfortable as possible to support his/her own healing potential. Aspirin (or acetoaminophen) should be given if fever or pain suggests that the child needs such a drug. The discomfort of the swollen parotid glands is often relieved by an icepack, or by the warmth of a heating pad or a hot-water bottle; ask the child what feels best. The discomfort of other affected glands is less directly treatable, although an icepack may be comforting for a swollen testicle. The headache of meningoencephalitis is often relieved by darkening the room that the child is resting in, and by quiet. Other remedies for headache (such as neck massage) should be offered.

The most direct remedy for mumps is prevention. Mumps vaccine may be given to any child after the age of 15 months. It is offered in a single injection, combined with vaccines for measles and German measles (rubella).

## Nosebleeds

Nosebleeds are rare in infancy but common in preadolescent children. A small blood vessel of the mucous membrane, usually in the forward part of the nose, becomes congested and then broken, leading to an outpouring of blood.

*Personal symptoms.* Sometimes nosebleeds are preceded by a bump to the child's face. Aside from nosebleeds that are set off by trauma, the three common conditions that lead to nosebleeds are:

- Some congestion of the blood vessels of the mucous membranes in the nose: a cold or a nasal allergy.
- Dryness of the air, as in the winter when the house heat is turned on.
- The child's picking his/her nose, thus causing a small blood vessel to break.


*Physical signs.* Blood can be seen running out of the child's nostril. Often some blood is swallowed which can cause vomiting (preceded by belly ache) and black or tar-colored stools.

*Other things you should know.* Nosebleeds rarely signal more serious dis-ease. If your child has as many as three nosebleeds in one week, and especially if both sides of the nose are bleeding, you will want to consider the possibility of high blood pressure (determined by taking the child's blood pressure), a bleeding tendency (indicated by multiple black-and-blue spots of unexplained cause, and sometimes by bleeding from other places in the body), and rheumatic fever (indicated by fever and the appearance of illness in the child).

*Remedies.* Most nosebleeds stop after a teaspoonful or so of blood has been lost. If the bleeding continues, or if it is at all brisk, use the following procedure:

- Have the child blow the nose vigorously. This is a very important step. A loose clot of blood, only partially attached, cannot seal over the blood vessels. Loose mucous also prevents a firm clot from forming. The nostril must be clear of all this material before a firm clot can form at the bleeding point.

- Have the child sit up and lean forward; pinch the nostrils together, firmly for ten minutes by the clock.

- Most nosebleeds will have stopped at this time; if the bleeding continues, repeat the procedure once.

- If the bleeding still continues, apply a little petroleum jelly to a small bit of cotton or gauze and wedge it firmly in the nostril; wait one half hour.

- If the nosebleed still continues (very few nosebleeds last beyond an hour) you will want to consult a professional so that the open blood vessel can be sealed by heat (cautery) and/or the nose can be packed using special instruments.

Once the nosebleed has stopped, remind the child that swallowed blood may give him/her a mild belly ache or a sense of nausea. This passes after the blood has been vomited or has moved from the stomach into the gut. Loose or black stools will end in a day or two.

One nosebleed leads to another. The clot that seals over the bleeding vessel dries to a scab and itches as it heals. The child — who usually has the same cold or allergic condition that caused congestion of the blood vessels of the nose in the first place — picks at the itchy scab, and another nosebleed starts. This event often happens when the child is asleep, and the nose-picking is quite involuntary. To prevent this sequence, run a cool-mist vaporizer in the room at night (to keep the mucous membranes of the nose from drying), put a little petroleum jelly in the nostrils — or let the child do it — and, if necessary, put socks over the hands or pin over the sleeves of the pajamas so s/he does not scratch at his/her nose while sleeping.

Offer a diet rich in iron-containing foods after a nosebleed. If the child has had several nosebleeds in a row, have the hematocrit checked; children often have a small iron reserve, and a little bleeding can cause an anemia (see section on Anemia).

## Roseola

Roseola is one of the fever/rash illnesses of childhood; it commonly occurs between the ages of 6 months and 3 years, and is presumably caused by a virus.

*Personal symptoms.* A high fever of sudden onset is the first indication of this illness. Except for the discomforts resulting from the fever, the baby shows no particular symptoms. When the fever is reduced to a point where it no longer causes discomfort for the baby, s/he seems entirely well, cheerful, not irritable, eats and drinks well, plays as usual, and is only a little more sleepy than usual.

Because the initial fever comes on so quickly and characteristically rises to such a high level (40.6°C/105°F by rectum is not uncommon) and because of the age of the child, this is often the occasion for a febrile convulsion (see section on Convulsion). Any child who has had a first convulsion should be seen and evaluated by a professional.

The incubation period for roseola is 1½ to 2 weeks. You may know that your baby was in contact with another child with this disease (mothers should be very careful to inform each other about such exposures) or you may never know where the exposure occurred. Presumably children are often exposed to contagious illnesses in public places like grocery stores.

*Physical signs.* The fever may be steady (that is, recurring at the previous high level after the effect of aspirin has worn off in four hours) or it may come and go. It usually lasts for one to four days. During this time there are almost no symptoms or signs of specific illness. There may be a mild runny nose. The throat may appear a little reddened. Nodes in the neck may be somewhat enlarged but usually do not seem to be tender. The nodes at the back of the juncture of the head and neck, at or just below the hairline (the occipital nodes) may be enlarged to the size of almonds; this is a characteristic sign of the illness.

Because of the usual age of the child who has this illness, you will want to be very careful to check repeatedly for indications of more serious or treatable disease. Examine the ears with an otoscope and watch the child thoughtfully for signs of earache: pulling on ears, crying unexplainably, pulling at hair, rubbing cheeks, or hitting the side of the head. Examine the neck to be sure that it bends forward easily and with no discomfort for the child. Notice whether the child seems to have discomfort when urinating — a possible indication of a urinary-tract infection. Examine the throat for significant redness or white patches, and watch the child carefully to note whether there seems to be any discomfort when s/he swallows, especially while eating solids. Look for cough and rapid or difficult breathing (remembering that breathing always speeds up when body temperature is very high, slowing again when the temperature is brought down closer to normal) and listen to the chest with a stethoscope.

After the fever has subsided — in one to four days — the child will break out in a rash. The rash may be very fleeting (seen before a nap, gone by the time s/he wakes up) or it may fade slowly over a day or two. The rash is fine, red, slightly raised, and turns pale on pressure, like a sunburn. It is most noticeable on the trunk, arms, and neck, and may or may not spread to the face and legs. It does not seem to itch.

*Other things you should know.* As with all contagious rash illnesses, the child should be considered contagious to others from a day or so before the fever begins (probably the most contagious period) until the rash has disappeared completely. Adults rarely have this illness, at least not in its characteristic form, but it is possible that any viral infection can affect a fetus in the first three months of intrauterine life. Caution anyone in contact with your ill baby — especially anyone who *might* be in the first few weeks of a pregnancy — about the contagiousness of the illness. There is no reason why the baby should not be outside in nice weather if s/he feels like playing outside, but it is irresponsible from a community-health point of view to take the child to a grocery store or playground where s/he will expose others to the illness. Prospective visitors to your house can be asked whether they want to risk exposure, and you should notify others whom you and the baby plan to visit.

Most will feel relaxed about exposure to so mild an illness, but the decision should be theirs to make.

There is no specific curative remedy for this viral illness. Sustain the child's self-healing with thoughtful offerings of nutritious food and some extra cuddling. Care for the child in the little comforting ways that reassure him/her that you are there.

Roseola is often the first serious illness a baby will have. It requires close attention to health assessment and physical examination, differentiation from other more threatening conditons, and closely attentive healing assistance. When your baby's roseola has come and gone and you have accomplished your role in healing at home with thoughtfulness and competence, you can feel justly proud. You will (as I do, always) feel very worried until your child's illness is over; competence in healing at home does not mean that you are unconcerned or totally self-confident!

## Rubella

Rubella, also called German measles or three-day measles, is a viral infection that is brief, not very incapacitating, and ends with a rash.

*Personal symptoms.* There is an incubation period of 2 to 3 weeks. The initial symptoms include mildly enlarged nodes in the neck, especially those behind the ears and at the base of the skull. There may be a runny nose. The illness generally begins with fever, although this is not necessarily very high. There are no specific complaints from the child, only the crankiness of feeling ill and the discomforts of fever.

*Physical signs.* Examination is nonspecific, except for the rash. It is red, slightly raised, and may itch. It generally begins on the face and the trunk and spreads downward.

*Other things you should know.* If a woman is pregnant and is not immune to rubella, she can contract the disease and her unborn child can experience it at the same time. For her the disease is mild. For her child-to-be rubella can cause serious problems: malformations of the heart, the eyes, and the brain. Apparently many viral infections can adversely affect the development of the fetus during the first few weeks of fetal development. The syndrome brought about by rubella virus is best known because it was studied after an identified epidemic in 1964.

Many viral infections cause a rubellalike illness — brief, mild, involving a fever and a rash. It is possible to identify rubella by sending two specimens of a patient's serum, taken a few weeks apart, to a research center. In most individual cases of fever-and-rash illness, however, we do not carry out these tests, and therefore we are often uncertain whether any single instance of viral fever-and-rash illness is rubella or not.

Immunization of every child against rubella (girls because they may at some time be pregnant, and boys because they could expose a pregnant woman to their rubella illness) is important — not because the illness of rubella is any particular hardship, but because this is one fetal hazard that can be prevented. It is also courteous to notify any woman of childbearing age who comes to visit your ill child that there is the danger of exposure to a viral illness; the most damage to the fetus is done at a time when many women are not yet certain they are pregnant. Only she can decide whether she wants to expose herself to an agent that might be damaging to her fetus.

*Remedies.* No specific remedy exists for rubella, nor is any called for. The illness is mild and brief, and one needs only to support the ill child, to comfort, and to offer assistance to the child's own healing capacities.

## Salicylism

Salicylism is the state of poisoning with a salicylate drug; its most common antecedent is an administered overdosage of aspirin.

*Personal symptoms.* Aspirin poisoning used to be far and away the most common poisoning of children. Since the introduction of safety caps for drug bottles, it is now a much less frequent occurrence for a child to find, open, and eat the contents of a bottle of aspirin. There remain, however, many instances in which a child is made ill by inadvertent overdosage of aspirin by a parent.

Like many drugs, aspirin has a fairly narrow margin between therapeutic effect and toxicity. It is often tempting to think that if two aspirin are the correct dose for a fever, four aspirin should be given for a very high fever. A child can easily become poisoned, especially a child who is already ill. S/he may become somewhat dehydrated because all healing energies are concentrated on the disease for which the aspirin is being given.

The initial symptoms of aspirin poisoning are deep respirations and sleepiness; there may be belly ache and vomiting. Other symptoms are ringing in the ears, dizziness, blurred vision, sweating, generalized numbness and tingling, and easy bleeding.

*Physical signs.* Breathing with increased depth but without increased rate can be recognized. Difficulty in rousing the child is usually the first sign that the child's illness has taken a new turn.

The most specific observations about aspirin poisoning are made by laboratory tests. If you suspect that your child has taken in an excess of aspirin, blood tests will measure the changes in dissolved salt and gas concentration that reflect the major hazards of aspirin poisoning. Aspirin poisoning, even in moderate degree, is a serious problem that requires hospitalization.

*Remedies.* The treatment for aspirin poisoning is primarily given by intravenous infusion of salts planned to combat and overcome the effects of too much aspirin in the bloodstream.

The most important remedy for this condition, of course, is preventive; do not exceed the recommended doses of aspirin.

### Splinters

A splinter is a small piece of foreign material (often wood or glass) embedded in the skin or under a nail.

*Personal symptoms.* If the child does not complain that the splinter hurts, there is usually no need to remove it. The body will work to expel the bit of foreign material. Check it occasionally to be sure that it has not become infected, if it does it can be treated at that time.

*Physical signs.* Most splinters can be removed at home. If you believe that a splinter entered the skin and you cannot see it, it may need to be checked by a profesional. If it is in the hand or the foot, in or near a joint, or anywhere on the head, it might cause damage if not removed. Similarly, a piece of metal traveling at high velocity might enter the abdominal cavity. Deeply imbedded splinters in muscle can probably be left alone, as the procedure for removal is itself not entirely benign. A deeply embedded splinter of metal or glass can be seen on X-ray.

*Remedies.* If the child agrees that the splinter hurts so much that s/he wants it removed, wash the surrounding skin well with Betadyne or pHisohex soap. Wipe a needle and tweezers with alcohol. Give the child some outrageous treat, like a piece of candy or gum. Use an ice cube to hold against the skin for quick and surprisingly effective topical anesthesia. Lift the end of the splinter with the needle and pull it out with the tweezers.

## Sprains

A sprain is a painful condition in which ligaments — the bands of connective tissue that hold the bones of a joint together — are pulled or stretched.

*Personal symptoms.* A sprain can be caused by a blow to a joint or can happen when the joint is stretched or twisted. Ankle sprains often occur when a child stumbles and twists the ankle.

Because the sprain is painful the child will guard the arm or leg and not want to move it as usual. S/he may also have noted that the joint that is hurting is somewhat swollen compared to the same joint on the other side. You will also want to ask whether the child heard a "pop" or "snap" when the injury occurred; for a very young child this question can only be answered by an observer. If this noise was heard there should be an X-ray examination to check for a broken bone.

*Physical signs.* When you examine the joint there will be tenderness and probably some swelling. If the swelling is very great the injury may be a broken bone and not just a simple sprain. Also, if the injured area is black and blue, if there is one place that is very, very tender, if the child refuses to move the joint at all, or you feel a crunchy sensation when you touch the joint firmly with your fingers, you will want to consult a professional to check for a fracture.

*Remedies.* The immediate pain of a sprained joint should be relieved by aspirin and a half hour of rest. If the child is still crying inconsolably you should reconsider the need for professional consultation.

Apply an icepack to the injured joint off and on for the first 24 hours. An icepack can be made by putting ice into a plastic bag, sealing it securely, and wrapping it in a towel. Remember that a young child who is not in very much pain will not want to sit still with an ice bag for long periods of time; the intent is to help the child to heal his/her body, not to make the child miserable.

Splint or protect the joint from movement for about 24 hours. You can make a sling to protect a wrist or elbow; an Ace bandage can be wrapped around an ankle or knee. Children heal so quickly that they may be fully active before the 24 hours have passed. You need not discourage a child from moving an injured joint — s/he will refuse to move it if it is very painful. A sling or Ace bandage can help the child avoid unnecessary but habitual movement. Unless the sprain is minimal, it will heal better if it is kept still for about a day.

After 24 hours, heat and massage will help the sprain heal. Both should be gentle and soothing and should feel good to the child.

Remember to offer the child an especially good diet to help the healing and suggest interesting things to do while s/he is sitting around waiting for the joint to feel better.

## Sunstroke and Heat Exhaustion

These two conditions, which may occur in mild or serious form, both result from prolonged exposure to hot sun.

*Personal symptoms.* The child will have been out in the sun for some time; that interval varies from one individual to another. In both conditions s/he will complain of weakness, and of feeling faint or dizzy and uncomfortable. S/he may collapse while playing. In heat exhaustion there may be muscle cramps and headache. With heat exhaustion, s/he will not have drunk enough salt-containing fluids to keep up with the sweating. With sunstroke, s/he will have overheated the body so that the normal temperature-regulating mechanism of the brain cannot keep body temperature down.

*Physical signs.* The child with heat exhaustion will feel cool and clammy to the touch; s/he will appear pale and sweaty. With sunstroke, the child will appear red and flushed, the skin will feel dry and not sweaty, and body temperature will be elevated.

*Remedies.* If the child has collapsed while playing, you should take him/her to an emergency room. If s/he has come in to rest, you may provide treatment at home unless body temperature is higher than 40.6°C/105°F, as in sunstroke. If the child does not look and feel better after an hour of home care, you should consult a professional by telephone for advice. If an infant under 2 years appears to have sunstroke or heat exhaustion, you should consult a professional immediately.

For heat exhaustion, the remedy is to offer salt and carbohydrate-containing fluids to drink. Allow the child to choose what sounds good and offer a variety of drinks. Have the child lie down with feet elevated.

For sunstroke, have the child lie down, undressed, or covered with a light sheet, and follow instructions for lowering fever (see section on Fever). Check the child's temperature every fifteen minutes. Do not give drinks designed to make him/her sweat — hot drinks, or drinks with ginger or cayenne.

## Teething

At about the age of 4 months, most babies enter a stage called
"cutting teeth." Each tooth actually cuts through the gums in
a matter of a few hours, but for weeks or months before this
babies appear to be affected in a variety of ways by teeth that
are working their way out. The stage lasts until the age of 2 or
2½ years.

*Personal symptoms.* Occasionally a two-year-old can indicate that his gums are painful. Mostly it is the observant and
experienced mother who guesses that the baby is troubled by
teething. Refusing to suck milk, refusing solids or being finicky
about foods, crying before going to sleep, waking in the night,
and general crankiness are common indicators that a baby is
unhappy because of the discomforts of teething.

*Physical signs.* Teething causes an increase in quantity
and quality of saliva. Teething babies drool and have perpet-
ually wet chins. They also swallow some of the extra saliva;
this can be irritating to the stomach so that the baby spits up
more than usual — often a mouthful of food or milk that is
slimy with mucous. The swallowed saliva can also come
through in the stool, producing a stool that is looser than usual,
full of mucous and with an acrid and distinctive smell. The
excess saliva can pool at the back of the throat and cause a
light cough that has the effect of clearing the throat.

Characteristically, the saliva of a teething baby contains a
substance that can be irritating to skin. It can cause a fine red
rash on the chin, neck, and upper chest if the baby is a drooler.
It sometimes causes a rash around the nipples of a nursing
mother. And commonly it causes a rash in the diaper area that
is bright red and looks almost like a scald; this rash can appear
a few moments after the baby has passed a stool.

Teething also seems to increase congestion of the mucous
membranes of the upper airway passages. The baby may have
a chronically stuffy nose. This congestion, which is similar to
that caused by allergy, seems to increase the baby's suscepti-
bility to upper respiratory infections — viral colds, ear infections, and so on. It is difficult to know by observing a baby

whether s/he is pulling at the ears because the gums hurt (and ears are easily found handles to pull on) or whether s/he has an earache.

Sometimes babies have fevers associated with teething. A fever that goes up and back down again in a matter of a few hours rarely means a serious infection, if the baby has no other symptoms of illness.

Teething symptoms usually are intermittent and do not go on at a serious or worrisome pitch for days and days. If crying, irritability, listlessness, vomiting (as opposed to spitting up, which means losing just a mouthful of food or milk), frequent diarrhea, ear-pulling, or head-shaking persist for as long as 36 hours, you should consult a professional. Teething rarely makes a baby look sick, just bothered.

*Other things you should know.* Our grandmothers knew a great deal about teething. There is little information on this subject to be found in pediatric textbooks. It is certainly a major cause for baby discomfort and for mother worry. Some babies appear to take teething in their stride. Others are quite miserable. Sometimes the first few teeth are bothersome, and later teeth erupt with little or no difficulty.

*Remedies.* Since pain is a major problem, aspirin is a standby remedy. However, if one were determined to overcome all the baby's pain it would be easy to fall into a schedule of giving aspirin every four hours for days and days. Aspirin given so regularly and so frequently has its own hazards of overdose, irritated stomach, and bleeding tendency. If you are giving aspirin for teething discomfort you should try to limit its use to once or twice in 24 hours. Give it when it is most needed — a half hour before bedtime for a baby who has trouble falling asleep, in the middle of the night for a baby who is wakeful and cannot seem to get back to sleep, or a half hour before feeding for a baby whose major difficulty is discomfort when sucking milk.

Sore gums are comforted by rubbing with your finger, and by the baby's chewing on something hard and cold. Carrot sticks (fat ones that will not break off in the baby's mouth and become a choking hazard) can be kept in the refrigerator for this purpose. So can some teething toys, but you must check carefully to be sure that there are no parts that can come off in the baby's mouth and no fluid-filled sections that can develop a leak and poison the baby if s/he swallows the fluid. A face cloth wrung out in icewater can be chewed on. For older babies, popsicles (made at home out of fruit juice) are comforting.

If a stuffy nose and a cough are really bothersome, an antihistamine may be helpful. Usually these troubles are more bothersome to parents than they are to the baby; treat the baby and not yourself. There is no particular good in trying to make a stuffy nose go away if it isn't any bother to the baby — in time it will clear by itself.

If skin rashes are serious, one can waterproof the baby's skin with ointments. Petroleum jelly in a thick layer should be tried first; other ointments containing zinc oxide (such as Desitin or Peri-Anal) offer the skin still more protection. Remember — especially for the diaper-area rash — that baby skin has a remarkable capacity to heal itself if left clean, dry, and exposed to air and light.

## Vomiting

Vomiting is the forceful expulsion by the stomach of its contents. Sometimes material from below the stomach (such as the greenish bile-stained secretions from the upper part of the small bowel) are also expelled.

*Personal symptoms.* In most cases, vomiting must be regarded as a protecting or healing response of the stomach to some condition of dis-ease. Vomiting commonly happens when there is an inflammation or infection of the gastrointestinal tract; when there is poison or some other disagreeable substance in the stomach (such as foods to which one has an allergy, or foods that are contaminated with bacteria); and when there is a blockage of the gastrointestinal tract below the stomach. Vomiting also occurs, by mechanisms that are not so clear-cut, with upper-respiratory infections, especially ear infections; with headache, central nervous system infections (meningitis and encephalitis), and brain injury (as after head trauma); with emotional upset; with infections of the urinary tract; and after violent or prolonged coughing. Vomiting also happens as a simple response to overfilling of the stomach

When a child begins to vomit, one should review the possibility of all of these reasons as explanation for the vomiting. Some persons vomit easily and readily; for some children vomiting is the first symptom of almost every new illness. Others feel nauseated and churning, but do not easily bring anything up. Still others rarely experience even an urge to vomit. Knowing your own child and his/her history of experience with illness will help you assess the meaning of an episode of vomiting.

Vomiting itself, while uncomfortable, is probably in most cases a helpful event. Once the stomach has been emptied, however, vomiting clear mucous or bile-stained intestinal contents probably accomplishes little in the healing process. In addition, if all subsequent fluid intake is returned as vomit the possibility of dehydration develops.

*Physical signs.* Examine the material that the child is vomiting; look for undigested food, which suggests that the stomach has been sitting as an immobile, inactive container since the last ingestion of food, thus indicating the time of onset of the dis-ease. Look for clear or bile-stained mucous. Black blood in vomitus indicates that the blood has been in the stomach for some time, and may have been swallowed, as from a nosebleed. Streaks of bright red blood are not uncommon after a child has vomited many times, and probably come from tiny superficial blood vessels in the stomach or esophagus that have ruptured with the strain of vomiting.

Unless the cause of the vomiting is readily evident, and if the vomiting happens more than once, examine the child in your ordinary routine. Look at the ears and throat; listen to the lungs; examine the belly for tenderness, and with a stethoscope for signs of obstruction; check the neck for stiffness and for enlarged nodes.

Check frequently, if vomiting continues, for indications of dehydration. A wet mouth with ample saliva is reassurance that the child is not yet dry. Notice how frequently the child is urinating and in what amounts. Feel the texture of the skin, especially the skin and subcutaneous tissue of the abdomen; with dehydration there is often a doughy, inelastic feel to these tissues.

If vomiting progresses to dehydration; if it persists past the point of emptying the stomach and you can find no reason, by considering recent events and by examining the child, to explain the vomiting; if there is significant belly pain, especially pain localized to one place; or if there is any sign of infection of the nervous system, the ears or throat, the lungs, or the urinary tract, you will want to consult a professional. Projectile vomiting, with great force, is always a reason for professional consultation.

*Remedies.* The first remedy is to leave the child alone until the stomach is emptied, waiting before you begin to offer any remedies. Most of us are grateful to be held while we vomit, and to have our faces wiped and our clothes changed if needed. Vomiting often is accompanied by great weakness, profuse sweating, and dizziness; help is needed.

When the stomach seems to have emptied itself, and if you have not discovered any reason to ask for professional help, begin by offering substances that will settle and calm the stomach. The first remedy to try is weak peppermint tea, sweetened with a little honey and offered warm or iced as the child prefers; a nursing infant will probably prefer this warmed. Only a sip should be taken at a time; after an interval of a few moments, to test the stomach's reaction, another sip can be taken. If the tea is vomited, wait 30 to 60 minutes and try again, more slowly this time. If this second dose of tea is also lost, try Coke syrup. Coke syrup, which is the concentrated liquid that fountains use to make Coke drinks, can be bought at most drugstores. One-half to one teaspoonful, given every ten minutes for an hour, will usually settle a stomach so that the vomiting stops, unless there is some reason for the vomiting that has nothing to do with the stomach.

When there has been no vomiting for an hour and a half, begin to offer the child clear liquids in small amounts. Clear liquids are liquids you can see through, including diluted fruit juices, weak broth, popsicles, sherbet made with water, and jellied fruit-juice mixtures. If you must, you can use commercial jellied dessert mixtures, fruit-juice preparations, and popsicles; many of these are overly sugared and contain potentially harmful dyes, however, and are better avoided if you can make and freeze popsicles and mix fruit juices at home. Herbal teas are also helpful. It is important to offer and try several alternative liquids, following the child's suggestions or indications of what seems to go down easily. Water is generally harder for an upset stomach to keep down than is water with something in it, such as diluted fruit juice. Since a major reason for this early feeding is the replacement of water, carbohydrates, and salts, it is evident that plain water is not usually the best substance for the child to drink.

The younger the child the sooner you will want to start to replace lost fluids; younger children have a larger proportion of water with dissolved salt than do older children, thus making the risk of dehydration greater. With older children one can wait hours before beginning to replace lost fluids.

The basic rule of thumb of feeding after a bout of vomiting is that if the stomach is filled with any large amount of anything, it is likely to empty itself again.

When there has been no vomiting for a period of from 4 hours (for a young infant) to 12 hours (for an adolescent) one can begin to offer nourishment again. This period of putting the stomach to rest by feeding it only mixtures of water, salts, and carbohydrates is essential for the healing of the stomach and cannot be rushed. It is important to recognize and admit that not feeding a child, especially when the child thinks s/he would like to eat something, is very hard for every mother to do.

The first feedings offered should be foods that are easily digested; avoid foods that are spiced, contain fat, and have undigestible fibers. Some standard first foods are boiled carrots, lean meats like chicken and veal, boiled rice, cooked cereals like cream of rice and cream of wheat, scraped raw apple, and dry soda crackers. Continue to offer clear liquids, and continue to urge small feedings, taken frequently and eaten slowly.

For infants under the age of 8 months, milk is still an important food even though milks (other than breast milk) usually contain significant amounts of fat and are avoided for the time being for an older child. After a four-hour period when there has been no vomiting, a breast-fed infant should be offered frequent small feedings of breast milk, alternating with the offer of additional clear-liquid feedings. (Incidentally, in the midst of an illness, one should not offer foods that the infant has not had prior experience with, with the exception of peppermint tea and apple juice, which rarely cause any upset to babies.) For infants fed on prepared formula, the regular formula should be offered in a dilution that is half-and-half with water — that is, formula made to its regular dilution and then additionally diluted by an equal volume of water. For infants fed cow's milk (evaporated, skim, or whole) a skim-milk formula should be made by bringing skim milk to a boil (which makes the milk protein more digestible) and then diluting half-and-half with water. Never feed boiled skim milk undiluted, for it contains a concentration of salt that is dangerous in the face of some degree of dehydration.

The duration of this stage of refeeding depends on how the child seems to feel. If there is no distress except for that of hunger, you can progress in the next feeding to a regular diet. If the child seems to be improving slowly, and if there is still no indication of a cause for the illness, you should proceed less quickly into a regular diet. In any case, the foods that you want to avoid until the child seems to feel entirely well are those that are very spicey, those that contain large amounts of indigestible fiber, and those with a high fat content, including ice cream, eggs, peanut butter and other butters, bacon, and other fatty meats.

Drugs that stop vomiting are not sufficiently safe for children, nor in ordinary instances is any drug needed. Most drugs that stop vomiting act on the brain.

See section on Diarrhea for a discussion of the management of vomiting when it occurs together with diarrhea.

# CHAPTER 6

# Nutrition, Relaxation, Exercise

"Preventive medicine" is a recent idea put forth by the government and medical-care establishment to combat criticism that there is too little concern for health as opposed to illness, and too much focus on the repair of distress and disability *after* they have occurred. Programs of preventive medicine usually argue that good health is the responsibility of the individual person. The notion that health should be the responsibility of the individual, however, includes two very dangerous corollary ideas. The first is that no larger group — not the community, not the government, not the society as a whole — should take a responsibility to insure the health of individuals. The second is that if you are sick it is your own fault, or, in the case of a child, the parent's fault.

Current preventive-medicine campaigns often blame the citizen for ill health and then exhort him/her to avoid activities and substances that endanger good health. These campaigns do not, so far, seem to be very successful. One reason for this is that little or no effort is being made to take the offending substance or activity away so that it ceases to be a health hazard. The offending substances and activities are almost always by-products of our industrial and consumerist technology. The World Health Organization now contends that at least 80 percent of all malignant cancers are caused by environmental poisons, and yet even our cancer researchers are not campaigning vigorously to decrease this constant poisoning faced by all of us. Automobiles are the immediate cause of a high proportion of all the serious injuries and accidental deaths suffered by our people, and yet massive subsidies have not been made available to build and distribute cheap and efficient bicycles with carrying devices for children, to create and protect bicycle routes, to develop simple forms of nonprivate transportation, and to reward the avoidance of automobile travel.

Another reason that preventive-medicine campaigns do not seem to be succeeding is that there are rarely any workable suggestions for alternative substances or activities that might replace the hazards exhorted against. This is particularly true when the activity or substance used is a matter of individual, private choice. We need not allow our children to watch violent shows on TV, but for many there is little other affordable entertainment. We need not let our children eat junk food that is high in calories and low in nutrition, but for many there is little or no available and affordable fresh, pesticide-free, and locally grown produce. Warnings against the hazards of a sedentary life devoid of vigorous physical exercise rarely are coupled with creative plans to shift the focus of physical-education programs away from competitive sports with star athletes and winning teams, toward truly educational programs that guide and encourage everyone to remain as accustomed as they were in their preteen years to the enjoyment of some kind of heart-pounding, panting exertion every day.

I also suspect that current so-called programs of public education in preventive medicine fail because most of us do not believe that representatives of the medical industry and of the government really care about our good health. The medical industry thrives on our distress, disability, dysfunction, and disfigurement. Nutritionists are sometimes in the pay of cereal companies. Drug experts who inform us about drug use are often connected to drug manufacturers. And practicing physicians have been taught that we — their patients — are not able to understand what they should be teaching us, and that we are too self-indulgent to care.

This dilemma may, in fact, be a salvation. Because experts and professionals have done such a poor job of reducing the health hazards that plague us, and because they know and care so little that our well-being is in such a sorry state, we clearly have to take these matters in hand for ourselves and for our children. We, individually and collectively, have the opportunity to manage one of the most important aspects of our life. We have the opportunity to invent, by our own careful thought and caring concern, our own patterns of healthful living.

The focus of *prevention* is largely one of avoidance — avoidance of the exposures that precipitate illness and injury. The focus of *health promotion*, on the other hand, is a positive reaching toward the pleasures of robust good feeling.

Nutrition, exercise, and relaxation are three areas of everyday activity that are central in the promotion of health. However, they represent only a beginning in that invented process. Does my child work and play with vigor and joy, with endurance and strength, with a solid sense of the value and beauty of self? What foods does s/he eat? What does my child eat that endangers her/his nutrition, now and in the future? What does s/he not eat that the body needs? How balanced is my child's intake over a period of a week or ten days? What does s/he see me eat? What does s/he see the other adults and children eating? Does my child now have eating habits that will carry her/him through a healthy life? Does s/he transport her/himself — walking, running, or by bicycle — so that s/he pushes muscular development? Does my child have and use opportunities for active and vigorous noncompetitive play, so that s/he flops down exhausted, sweaty, and happy? When my child is tense and anxious does s/he know how to heal his/her body — can s/he retreat into a state of relaxation, or go to someone else for a lap sit or a back rub or ask to be held?

There are, undoubtedly, other areas of health promotion. Nutrition, exercise, and relaxation are only first steps in the invention and practice of good health.

## Nutrition

The basic principle of good nutrition for children is simple to describe, if difficult to allow in the way we now live. Children have a remarkable ability to self-select a healthful and nutritionally sound diet, if they are offered a variety of healthful foods from which to make their selection.

Our major difficulty in providing good nutrition for children is to find and afford the good foods that they must have to select from. Our stores, schools, neighbors' homes, and places of recreation are flooded with foods that are far from optimally healthful. We are a malnourished nation. Many of us suffer from anemia, obesity, the protein and nutrient deficiencies of poverty, and the hazards of food additives and chemical substitutes for food. Our treated soils and sprayed crops may well be returning less nourishing produce than we hope. Centralized farming and widespread distribution bring us food that has lost, over storage and travel time, much of the nourishment it once had. We may be depleting rather than replenishing body stores as we consume foods that are refined, processed, and fortified. Even now we do not know enough about nutritional needs to be able to process artificial foods with confidence. Not too many years ago, an infant formula was constructed that was thought to contain every nutrient needed by a human baby. Most infants fed this manufactured formula appeared to do well. But a very few developed severe and protracted seizures. Painstakingly, it was discovered that the formula was lacking in trace amounts of a B vitamin, later called pyridoxine, and for those few infants that minute vitamin deficiency precipitated seizure activity in the central nervous system. We now know that pyridoxine is a vitamin that is not abundant in our diet, that deficiencies affect not only the central nervous system but also the skin, one's resistance to stress, and the metabolism of proteins and fats. All of the babies fed that artificial formula were at risk of chronic and subtle health problems; those few with their peculiar metabolic reaction of seizures were the tip of an iceberg.

In order to provide healthful foods for our children to choose from, we must, first of all, find places to purchase them.

Unrefined grains and flours, pesticide-free and fresh produce, unprocessed legumes, fruits and nuts, and additive-free dairy products and baked goods *are* available to most of us — by traveling long distances, by ordering through mail-order supply houses, by growing our own summer gardens and freezing or canning the harvest. But such foods are expensive and time-consuming to prepare.

Probably few of us can afford either the time or the money to feed our children nothing but the most healthful foods. In addition, as they go out in the world and are attracted by social pressures to the whole range of junk foods, they will be tempted to experiment with their own diets in the company of their friends. One cannot simultaneously honor a child's right to decide what food goes into his or her mouth, and guarantee that the child's diet is superbly nutritious. Feeding children thus becomes a compromise of good sense.

For instance, we know that many foods that are inexpensive are also relatively nonnutritious. They are less satisfying, and often give a high proportion of calories to nutrients. Because they are less satisfying, we are inclined to eat more of them. This increases the risk of obesity, as too many calories are ingested. It has been suggested that we solve both these problems by planning to pay twice as much for the food that we buy and to enjoy it twice as much while eating only half as much.

I strongly urge every mother to examine and reassess her own personal eating habits. Each of us is the one most constant influence in our children's lives. What we do, and how we feel about ourselves, has — for better or worse — an overbearing influence on the child. What *you* enjoy preparing and enjoy eating, matched with your vigor and sense of healthiness, will in the end constitute your child's most important lessons in nutrition.

*Feeding infants.* There is no question that breast milk is the most nutritionally excellent food for small infants. It is so digestible that breast-fed babies often have fewer and smaller stools than babies fed other kinds of milks. Although breast milk has a small amount of iron in it, that iron is so well absorbed that babies fed only breast milk until the age of 16 months still maintain their iron stores and hemoglobin levels. In addition, breast milk does not inhibit the absorption of iron from other foods as much as cows' milk does. Babies on breast milk also seem less at risk of early obesity.

A diet of milk alone is relatively deficient in vitamins A and C. In moderate climates where there is relatively little direct exposure to the sun's rays, everyone whose bones are still young and growing needs some dietary vitamin D. For these reasons infants fed breast milk or a cows' milk formula are usually offered a daily supplement of an ACD vitamin preparation. Alternatively, the A and D may be given in cod-liver oil and the vitamin C in fresh orange juice (strained and diluted, one part water to two parts juice) or in rose-hip tea. Most babies will drink two to four ounces of one or the other drink once a day, which is sufficient.

Solids need not be offered early for nutritional reasons if the baby is drinking breast milk. However, if the baby is not fed breast milk s/he should start eating some solids at about two months: rice cereal (which has iron in it), pureed apple-sauce, and mashed fresh bananas are some foods that are well tolerated by babies at this age. Applesauce tends to loosen a baby's stools, and bananas tend to firm them, so you can decide on the best balance for your child. An adult may get bored feeding this limited variety of foods to a small baby, but babies seem quite content to eat the same well-digested foods every day. Mashed yellow vegetables can be added next, followed by the dark green vegetables and meats at about 4 months. Dark green vegetables and meats are sources of iron, and by 4 months a baby's bone marrow is able to make hemoglobin, so it is important to be ready to offer these foods at about this age.

A small, inexpensive, hand-operated food mill (or an electric mixer, blender, or processer) will allow you to cook fresh foods for yourself and others in the household and serve some to the baby. Baby food in jars is probably less nutritious than food freshly prepared. Leftover amounts can be frozen in ice-cube trays, but should be served in about a week.

Remember to salt your baby's food lightly or not at all. Because high salt intake (actually, sodium intake) can potentiate high blood pressure, we would all — even infants — do well to limit the amount of salt we use. It is simply easier never to become accustomed to salty foods. Also, before the age of 4 to 5 months the infant's kidneys are too immature to handle a large salt load.

By about 5 months, babies begin to handle foods that are not completely smooth in texture. Ordinary table foods that can be cooked until soft or mashed can then be served — foods like regular adult oatmeal and other cooked cereals, cooked vegetables such as carrots, squash, potatoes, legumes like lentils and other beans, and meats that can be chopped fine such as chicken, fish, and tender roasts.

In families with a history of allergy, some foods should be postponed until near the end of the first year: wheat, berries such as strawberries, citrus fruits, eggs, and shellfish are among the foods that commonly bring on allergic reactions.

For breast-fed babies the primary reason to offer solids before the first birthday is that sometime around that age babies get very firm in some food preferences and are delighted with their power to refuse foods. It seems easiest to start some solids at the age when the baby *wants* to taste adult food — generally around 5 or 6 months.

Apparently any mammal can easily and quickly become addicted to sweet-tasting foods. Even breast-fed babies, offered cow's milk sweetened with syrup, quickly learn to prefer the sweeter taste and may even refuse the breast milk. Certainly before the time when our children go out of the house on their own we can control that inevitable introduction to sweets. The avoidance of sweet foods and a very limited use of refined sugar at the family table will forestall and may even effectively discourage the adoption of the idea that sweets are the best foods. As always, we adults must consider our own eating habits and their influence on our children. If we consider sweets to be the most pleasurable foods we can easily teach this addiction to our children by example. That addiction is also fairly easy to overcome. Most people report that if they do not eat sweet foods for a period of six months or so, they no longer crave them or even enjoy them very much. It is best for our children if we never — or almost never — have sweets in the house. It is then more likely that when a child is old enough to spend pocket money at the corner store there will be only a brief investigation of candies and other refined-sugar sweets.

*Feeding older children.* By 18 months most children can share meals with other members of the household and feed themselves after a fashion, thus exerting control over what goes into their mouths. It is difficult, perhaps even impossible — and certainly unwise — to spoonfeed a child after this time except as an occasional and special kind of loving gesture. This was approximately the age at which children in the nutritionists' studies self-selected their own excellently nutritious diets.

Lifelong eating habits — like many other kinds of habits of daily living — begin to be set at this age. Eating is a much-repeated event. Physical satisfactions, sensuous pleasures — even the notion of food as a reward — begin to solidify as familiar attachments to eating. So too, punishments like scoldings, forced feeding as retribution for being bad, and the attitude of "I don't care whether you like it, it's good for you" can become habitually associated with eating. Mothers control the ambience of mealtimes. If others at the table repeatedly create an atmosphere of stress and displeasure, it would be well to feed the toddler only with yourself and those in the household who find mealtime a time of contentment.

The self-selecting babies in the research projects created a nutritious diet over periods of one to two weeks. An individual child might eat nothing but carrot sticks at one meal, and nothing but bananas at another. For this reason it is sensible to put out a variety of foods, including some that you are certain are liked by each child. This does not mean extra cooking — foods like peanut butter, nuts and raisins, cottage cheese, yogurt and fruit, hard-boiled eggs, and whole-grain bread can be added to any meal with very little extra effort. A child should understand that s/he is encouraged to eat what sounds good, that the body is "smart" and can tell the child what it needs, and that s/he will probably want some of every kind of food over a period of a week or so. Preschool children, who enjoy categorizing as a mental game, quickly learn to enjoy the exercise of grouping foods into categories: meat is like chicken is like fish is like eggs; cheese is like yogurt is like cottage cheese is like milk; squash is like carrots is like sweet potatoes is like yams, and so on.

Many mothers allow older children *not* to eat one pre-pared food at any major meal; there might be a cooked vege-table dish and a bowl of mixed raw vegetables, from which a child could select a reasonable portion of one or the other. Most young children, incidentally, dislike mixed foods; they seem to prefer to be able to identify exactly what is going into their mouths. They often prefer vegetables uncooked rather than cooked — even vegetables that are not often served un-cooked, like broccoli and brussels sprouts. Preschool children also have relatively little muscle power in their jaws and may refuse meats like steak and roasts because they are too hard to chew, but may enjoy those same meats if they are chopped into small bits.

Most of us eat much more meat than we ought to, except, of course, the poor, who cannot afford to buy much meat. Those who are not vegetarian do well on two servings of meat weekly, although this may seem depriving to some adults. Meat is expensive and also extravagant of the world's re-sources, since it is much more costly to produce protein by passing vegetable materials through the body of an animal than it is for us to use vegetable sources of protein directly. The iron and protein that we get from meat we can also get from dairy products and especially from legumes — dried beans of various kinds. Vegetable protein is more available to us — better absorbed and utilized — when eaten with other specific kinds of foods. Every major meal should have some grains (dark bread or brown rice, for instance), some dairy products (cottage cheese or yogurt, for instance), some nuts and seeds (peanut butter or sesame seeds, for instance), some legumes (roasted soybeans or stewed navy beans, for instance), some vegetables (including those with dark green leaves), and some dried fruits (raisins and prunes, for instance). Even when a standard menu is served, all of these foods can appear as salad ingredients to select from. They can also be blended into salad dressings or dips, which children enjoy with raw vegetables — they enjoy the messiness of the process as much as the taste, I suspect.

Evidence is accumulating that we can be protected against a variety of bowel troubles, including appendicitis and bowel cancer, if we eat large amounts of vegetable fiber. This vegetable fiber is digested partly or not at all and causes bowel movements to be large in volume. Vegetable fibers are found in whole-grain foods and especially in raw fruits and vegetables, particularly in peelings, seeds, and cores.

In the midst of all of this nutritional good sense, mothers have to contend with advertising and the habits of their own generation. While most children like whole-grain bread if they have never eaten anything else and there is no white bread in the house, many adults and older children do not like dark breads and insist that some white bread be purchased or baked. Experiment with lighter dark breads and read ingredients labels; some whole-grain content is better than none at all. Some adults feel deprived if they do not have meat at every dinner meal; cook a small amount, be sure that there are other sources of protein and iron served, and do not force children to eat meat if they do not choose to. Some standard children's treats, like Spaghettio's, can be served now and then with the understanding that that sort of food doesn't do much for your body or your spirit. Absolute strictness about what foods are allowed, in the face of our prevailing cultural notions about food, is likely only to mean that the child will later go through a junk-food binge when s/he is old enough to eat away from the household. Every ordinarily curious child is going to want to know what those addictions to junk food are all about.

What foods should be absolutely avoided? I think the following list should be strongly discouraged — not "because I say so," but for the very clear reasons that they are hazardous to our health and to our enjoyment and appreciation of our bodies. They should be so strongly discouraged that they have little or no appeal for the child.

- Foods with artificial red dyes and other additives that are nutritionally nonnecessary and possibly harmful.
- Heavily salted foods like chips, because high salt intake is not a good habit.
- Foods made with artificial substitutes, many of which are addictive and harmful. An example of this is food that tastes sweet but is made with a (possibly harmful) sugar-substitute chemical.
- Foods that are almost entirely artificial, like "space bars." We were meant to eat foods from the earth, and such creations are fit only for machines. Nutritionists tell us that we as a nation have learned to prefer the tastes of "instant" or "processed" foods over the tastes of foods in their more natural state. It is difficult to think of any benefit to children in learning to prefer the tastes of artificial foodstuffs over those of real foods.

*Diet and disease prevention.* What about diet and the prevention of disease? There are as many individual ideal diets as there are individual constitutions. Each of us needs to learn, by trial and error, what balance of foodstuffs seems to keep us well. One person may need a high daily intake of vitamin C to escape respiratory infections, another may need extra magnesium-containing foods to avert temper tantrums, while another may ward off urinary-tract infections by drinking cranberry juice every day.

From the studies on self-selected diets, and from my own observations of children recovering from diseases of salt loss (such as severe diarrhea or vomiting, when losses of specific salts can throw the body chemistry out of balance) it seems clear that our bodies can tell us, through our appetites and cravings, what specific foodstuffs we need. Children are usually very keen to the demands of their bodies, being not yet socialized to know what most people do or what they are expected to do. Children should be urged, exhorted, and re-

warded for attending to these subtle signals. If there are cranberry juice, oranges, and bananas in the house for a snack, let
the child choose which s/he prefers but ask the child to do that
by listening to what the body says it wants. As adults, we can
recapture some of that body-signal attention, but it requires a
considerable effort and a filtering out of what we think we
*should* want to eat.

- Sugar intake. Excesses of refined sugar cause a sudden and
  extreme rise in blood sugar — the basis for the feeling of
  an energy surge. The body reacts to this high level of blood
  sugar by calling forth all mechanisms for lowering blood
  sugar as quickly as possible. The blood sugar thus drops
  fairly quickly, often to relatively low levels. The body then
  signals that it is deprived of sugar, and one feels a need
  for another feed of sugar. This cycling produces the common daily pattern of a sugary breakfast, a sugary mid-
  morning snack, a dessert food at noontime, a sugary after-
  noon snack, and so on through the day.

  There are several obvious health consequences of this
  pattern of eating. Sugar is high in calories, and the other
  foodstuffs that are usually combined with sugar — flour,
  butter or other fats and oils, chocolate, and so on — are
  also high in calories. Excess calories will be stored by the
  body as fat. Also, sugar has no nutritional value — it only
  provides a quick burst of energy, which, as we have seen,
  the body soon disposes of. A diet high in sugar discourages
  the eating of foods that give us long-lasting energy, because a sudden high-calorie load makes us feel satisfied.
  The body's blood-sugar reducing capacity is put to a great
  deal of strain in these repeated efforts of sudden and maximum mobilization. Some scientists believe that most if
  not all of us can become diabetic if we live long enough
  to exhaust the capacity of the pancreas (the organ that
  makes insulin, a major substance in the body's metabolism
  of sugar in the blood). Some of us, of course, are also
  particularly disposed to become diabetic by family history
  or by individual constitution.

  It seems logical that we can protect and preserve our

bodies' capacities by avoiding excessive dietary habits. In this case, the ordinary U.S. diet of 120 pounds of sugar a year (for each of us!) is clearly excessive; our sturdy pioneer foremothers and forefathers, for instance, consumed only 4 pounds of sugar per person per year in 1700. We have been taught this addiction by commercial interests playing on our natural mammalian tendency to a sweet tooth, but we can easily teach ourselves to undo that addiction. More importantly, we can arrange our in-household eating so that our children need never learn that that addiction is natural, to be expected, or a good thing.

• Salt intake. Similarly, we are accustomed to eating large amounts of table salt, sodium chloride. The sodium is excreted by our kidneys. A high blood load of sodium makes our kidneys work so hard that they send signals to the hormone system and blood pressure may increase. Possibly, as with diabetes, all of us can push our blood pressure up by eating, regularly, large quantities of sodium-chloride salt. Those of us with family histories of high blood pressure, or with an early propensity to a slightly high blood pressure (discovered at the regularly scheduled health assessments) are probably more susceptible than others to the effects of a high salt intake.

High blood pressure puts an extra load on the heart and probably increases the possibility of a heart attack. It also increases the possibility of hemorrhage (bleeding) from the blow-out of small vessels as the result of excessive pressure inside the vessel. When such a blow-out occurs in the brain it is called a "stroke" or a "shock."

These are problems of middle or later age, but they are processes that begin in infancy. Avoidance of these later difficulties begins with appetites that are accustomed to lightly salted foods. We do of course need some sodium in our diets; we get some in most of the foods that we eat, even with no added salt. At times — for instance when we sweat a lot, or when we vomit or have diarrhea — we may need more salt, according to the signals our bodies give us.

For those of us accustomed to eating heavily salted food, it is a wonder to discover how foods taste different, and more interesting, without salt. For those of us who have to wean ourselves away from salt, the liberal use of other seasonings — garlic, lemon juice, herbs, and the various peppers — gives food that is strongly flavored but not salty. As always, our children follow our habits; most children who routinely use a saltshaker at the beginning of a meal have seen this done by one of the adults in the household.

- Cholesterol intake. Foods that help the body to make or retain high levels of cholesterol — notably eggs, animal fats (like meat fat and butter), and other saturated fats — predispose to heart attacks by increasing the possibility that the blood vessels will be lined with deposits of cholesterol. This process happens to many of us, and for those who have this propensity the process can begin in early childhood. In some families there is a metabolic tendency to carry high levels of fats in the blood (hyperlipidemia); others, of course, can have this condition with no family history.

  In families with a history of early (before age 45) heart attacks, a history of familial high blood pressure, or a history of hyperlipidemia, I would urge careful restriction of cholesterol-potentiating foods. For the rest of us, I usually advise a much more moderate course: unsaturated fats for all cooking where the flavor of saturated fats is not important, limited table use of butter if the family prefers that to margarine, limited consumption of meat fat except for those individuals who seem to crave it and who may perhaps need it. Eggs are a fine source of protein, a favorite food of most children, and a cheap and natural foodstuff, despite the fact that standard feeding and processing technology make eggs less nutritious than they might be. I would not urge any limitation in egg consumption for children unless specific health reasons dictate.

- Vitamins. What about vitamin supplements for children who have attained an adultlike diet (usually at 18 months)? There are certain circumstances when it seems reasonable and even necessary to use vitamin supplements, in pill, chewable tablet, or liquid form.

One circumstance is when a child is going through a period of food finickyness and it seems important not to get into a contest of wills. Children commonly use mealtime disputes about what foods will and will not be eaten as a way of testing for more personal autonomy. Tests of personal autonomy are important developmental steps, and must be allowed to play themselves out. At the same time, we never want a child to get trapped into eating a poor diet as a consequence of such a test. It is often a good idea, then, to give some daily multivitamin supplement and stop arguing with the child over food consumption, knowing that when the pressure is off the child will probably return promptly to a new version of a previously well-balanced diet.

Another time for vitamin supplementation is during recovery from disease. When a child is having a *slow* recovery from an illness, the body needs, for immediate and daily use, a superbly nutritious intake. When a child has a *series* of illnesses, however small and inconsequential, vitamin supplementation is also advised. Repeated bouts of illness make drains on our reserves as we heal ourselves; if those reserves are not to be depleted we need an especially good diet to counteract the drains. When a child has had a series of illnesses the appetite often flags and s/he may feel cranky enough to fall into arguments about what foods will be eaten.

It is also true that children are small creatures and all of their body reserves are smaller in absolute quantity than those of adults. They can be depleted rather quickly, even in the course of a single illness, and the depletion can predispose the child to other illnesses. Daily-minimum-requirement doses of vitamins and minerals will not be harmful and might resolve a problem of illness-susceptibility.

We also discover, by trial and error, special and individual vitamin needs. It is probably true that some of us need high daily amounts of vitamin C to ward off respiratory ailments and cannot get those amounts in ordinary foods. While I would prefer that children be allowed to follow their appetites on such needs and eat the foods that will bring them, in a natural form, the vitamins that they need, I would never argue with a parent who says, "When I give her 100 mg of vitamin C she doesn't get colds, and when she doesn't take it she gets every cold that's going around."

For some people, the best and most rapid remedy for severe anxiety is a single large dose of B vitamins. This preparation is marketed commercially as Stress-tabs. It is a useful preparation for a child who is acutely frightened, in pain, or upset for other reasons.

I am clearly out of step with many who have analyzed our dietary habits and advise that everyone take vitamin supplements every day. I am convinced that if we have nutritious food from which to choose, barring individual special needs, we are better off getting our nourishment from natural sources than from the use of manufactured chemicals. The vitamin industry is big business, geared to make profits like any other big business. Heavy and routine use of any commercial supplemental nonfood is not right for good health.

I also worry that children will get a message that they can eat any junk foods they want as long as they take their daily vitamin pill. As with the infant formulas, I suspect that even multiple vitamin and mineral supplements do not have substances that we need for good health.

- Special foods. There are certain foods that recur in many cultures and over many generations as special sources of healthiness. I think that we ignore this sort of folk wisdom at our own peril. These foods are thought to be especially good for us to sustain good health and to enable us to repair the ravages of everyday experience. I include them as part of a disease preventing diet because they are so easily worked into our diets on an almost daily basis with little cost or inconvenience, and with a comfortable assumption that we are feeding ourselves well.

These foods are lemons, garlic, onions, cabbages, and carrots. Each has a history and lore of special disease-preventive and healing properties. This lore has for the most part not been substantiated by research evidence — perhaps because researchers have not asked the right questions. These foods are all highly nutritious, and a child can eat them as often as possible for good health.

Our children's adventures with the foods they eat are funny. One great frustration is to invest money and effort and time in preparing something that is then refused or eaten only with distaste. The vagaries of children's appetites, their avid enjoyment of a food one week followed by vehement dislike the next week, the self-importance and pride in their pronouncements about "what I need," their vigorous efforts to learn about themselves and their fantasies about the inner workings of their own bodies — all of these are wonderful and delightful if only we can see the funny side of their struggles with themselves and with us. For me, always, the humor is best savored when it is shared with other mothers.

## Relaxation

Good health demands the effective balance of two complex, whole-person processes that are closely related to each other. The first of these is moving and acting, focusing one's energy and strength, responding to challenge and initiating sustained and directed effort. The second is regenerative rest, the easing of mind, spirit, and body.

Our Western philosophy has clouded the understanding that these processes are integrally related to each other. Emphasis on achievement and especially on the *products* of achievement has clouded our understanding and appreciation that effective, outward-directed energy must push off against an even serenity and a centering of unattached energy. Exertion and restorative repose must be seen, in the illumination of an

understanding of healthiness, as interrelated, mutually inter-
twined, and in balance.

Both of these processes involve thinking, feeling, and muscular and nervous adjustments that are often, for adults, outside of our ken. In many ways children are more attuned to
these interconnections. Watch a small child asleep, or sitting
on a rock dreamily picking his/her toes, or charging about in
active and strenuous play. One senses that all facets of the
person are in harmony; there is no reserve, disengagement, or
alienation. For all of their lack of experience, our children can
teach us much about these matters. And from our experience,
we adults can guide our children — if we can comprehend
what we have learned about ourselves.

*Stress and the stress response.* The stress response is initiated by stressors, signals that we perceive as calling forth
exertion. For effective coping we need to be able to harness the
stress response, the physiological and psychological whole-
body state that gears us to efficient and forceful activity. But
a constant state of stress, with an inability to regenerate by
relaxation when the stress response is inappropriate or at the
end of focused exertion, diminishes our effectiveness when we
need to be effective. Indeed, a persistent stress response that
is not or cannot be turned to effective action can drain the
physical and spiritual self and can even produce distress, dysfunction, and other signs of dis-ease.

The stress response, which galvanizes us into action, is a
physiological and psychological set for a variety of efforts that
serve as coping mechanisms. These coping mechanisms can
be harnessed defensively, to ward off or overcome danger, or
creatively, to generate change, productive achievement, and
flights of inventive growth.

The stress response increases the rate and volume of our
heart's beat, tones our blood pressure, and reduces the blood
flow in our innards and extremities so that the supply of oxygen, sugar, and other nutrients to our large muscles, brain, and
cardiovascular system can be increased. A variety of hormones
are released in minute but very effective amounts to alert and

tune sensory perception, awareness of external events, muscular tension, metabolic rate, and rapid and efficient breathing.

Infants produce a stress response that is undifferentiated and unmodulated. The stressors that they perceive are only signals for alarm; there is too little experience to distinguish between danger and simple discomfort, too little integrative intelligence to cope constructively, too much dependence to initiate creative action. In infancy this holistic response is triggered by hunger, physical discomfort like wetness or cold, a lack of comfortable and comforting support — being undressed, being in a tub of water, or being held with fear, anxiety, anger, or disgust.

After about four months, there are more discerning differentiations of the nature of the situation to which the infant reacts. Cries of hunger, frustration, and pain gradually become distinguishably different. As the child learns to move around in space — to creep, crawl, and then walk — there are increasingly effective exertions: get to that rattle, pull that cloth off the table, pick up those bits of cereal.

Throughout childhood we learn when and how to be alarmed and how to react effectively. We also learn to recognize situations in which strenuous exertion will bring the rewards of achievement, accomplishment, and glorious imaginative creation. Adults have words for these perceptions and these responses. With words it is possible to refine perceptions, to understand that fear and anger have different antecedents and call for different responses, and to bask in appreciation of our energies and accomplishments.

If my child looks wan or sad, or thrashes about protestingly, or is frozen tense, I need to notice what has been happening and to think about signals for her sadness or anger or fear. I can recognize her adaptive stress response when her coping activity is effective. I want to help her become aware of these and also of her less effective stress responses, to name and learn alternatives. I can only start her on the road to self-understanding. Soon she will outstrip me in her understanding of her self. Her insights may help me as I struggle to understand myself better.

Together, mother and child, we explore the interconnections between toning exercise, exertional stress, and relaxation. As with the individual idiosyncracies of biochemical nutrition, each of us has individual needs and modes of toning and of repose. My ways are not my child's ways, but there are parallels. And the sensuous pleasures of exertion and accomplishment, of relaxation and restoration, are worthy of parallel appreciation.

*Stress and dis-ease.* When the stress response is adaptive, forcused, and effective it is a prime example of good health in action. When it is inappropriate, unrecognized, and diffuse we can feel sick or make ourselves sickness-prone. The child who fears leaving home to go to school may have real and significant abdominal pain, a poor appetite, and diarrhea; not only is the child not using her/his potential for good health, s/he is also suffering a kind of dis-ease.

The drained, frustrated energy that goes into chronic stress responses, to stressors that we don't even recognize or can't acknowledge, absorbs the defenses we ordinarily have on reserve to deal with exposure to infections, injuries, and so on. There is a growing body of evidence that a chronic state of stress can cause a variety of dis-ease states like high blood pressure, peptic ulcer, excess secretion of thyroid hormone, spastic or nervous gut (with diarrhea, vomiting, and/or belly ache), skin rashes, arthritis, and allergic reactions. In this way a vicious cycle is set up in which chronic unidentified stress leads to significant dysfunction, which in turn further reduces the effectiveness of our coping and our defenses for resisting threats to healthful functioning.

Learning to deal with stress is thus a major and critical aspect of both the prevention of dis-ease and the promotion of health. We must help our children learn to maximize the effectiveness of the stress response and to harness its energy. We need to help them identify the subtle toll taken when that energy is wasted, learn to know their personal stressors, and integrate thought, feeling, and physiologic response in order to minimize wasteful stress response and maximize directed and effective stress response. Learning to deal with stress also means learning how to relax.

*How to relax.* Relaxation is more than a state of muscles: it is also a state of mind and spirit. Relaxation is intensely pleasurable. We begin our lives with a facility for complete and intense relaxation. Watch a child falling asleep. If it is your child, and if you are in tune, you can almost feel in your own body the loosening of tension and the suffused ease.

As children grow older they begin to hear messages from the dominant culture about the value and virtue of relaxation and their entitlement to it. They hear that:

- Being productive (making, achieving, accomplishing) is the most highly valued, the most approved activity.
- Staring into space and daydreaming are somewhat shameful activities, oftentimes allowed only in the privacy of one's own space.
- The sensual enjoyment of relaxation is a pleasure for which one must pay with work, apologies, or suffering. These messages come not only from mothers. Some mothers even assiduously avoid teaching these dominant values. But they *are* dominant cultural values, and they do spoil, if not absolutely destroy, that innate childish capacity for total, self-absorbed relaxation.

And yet, as we all intuitively know, serene relaxation must alternate with vigorous exertion. Not only is the efficiency of the physical exertion at stake, but also the collected peacefulness of mind and spirit that is necessary for organized, planned, and sustained exertion and accomplishment. And we might, if we valued and respected our selves, count relaxation as important in our daily experience as accomplishment.

Only we can know, for our selves, the frequency, duration, and depth of relaxation that we need at any given moment. The state of relaxation needed and desired at any point in time depends on the degree and kind of exertion of the period immediately prior, the exertions that we expect to be demanded in the near or distant future, and the current overarching worries, demands, puzzles, and predicaments of our lives. I cannot legitimately say to my child, "You have rested enough, now" — although I can explain that the economy of our household demands that she finish cleaning her room, now, so that I can launder her clothes in preparation for the upcoming school week!

For each of us there are, also, good and not-so-good ways to find peace in relaxation. I am impressed when I talk to older children — in the preteen and teen years — about their evident need for more and more satisfying periods of relaxation in their day. They rarely can tell themselves or me how it is that they do find relaxation. Tension headaches are common for children in these years. After a thorough history and physical examination have ruled out other illness-related causes for the headaches, we talk about sources of stress in the child's life and ways to ease that stress by relaxation. I am not surprised that children of this age are relatively inarticulate about the stresses they are experiencing, but I am astonished that they cannot say what kinds of relaxation make them feel good. I do not believe that it is necessary, in the course of progressing through childhood, for a child to lose touch with that capacity for total and unself-conscious relaxation that was evident before s/he was "socialized."

There are a variety of techniques for relaxation. Some have become formalized, and there is a whole vocabulary for concepts, skills, and body parts. Some are taught, in classes or privately, by experts with various credentials. Some people feel good about learning from experts because they know that they care about themselves when they pay the fee. It is, however, unfortunate that we first destroy a child's innate capacity for self-knowledge and self-exploration, teach that the need for and the self-understanding of relaxation are invalid, and then offer professional services for the recapturing of what we need never have lost!

What follows are sketches of some of the most common and useful principles of the relaxation techniques. They are included to remind us, as mothers, that our children do begin by knowing how to relax. We can help preserve and expand this self-knowledge by applauding, explaining, putting words to, suggesting alternatives, and sharing with the child.

*The Relaxation Response.* Probably the simplest, most generally useful mode of relaxation is the so-called relaxation response. It consists of four essentials:

- Finding a quiet place as free as possible from distractions to the eye, ear, and senses of touch.
- Assuming a loose position in or on a comfortable bed, cot, mat, or chair.
- Taking on a passive attitude of letting things be as they are, ignoring both memories of unfinished happenings and forethoughts of the future.
- Repeating some simple sound or word, thus overcoming distracting sensations, pressing puzzles and plans, and the urge to do something.

Adults with high blood pressure who learn and perform this relaxation response twice a day for twenty minutes can drop their blood pressure by an average of five points, a significant change. Children past the age of 6 can relax intentionally in this manner and talk about what they are doing. Younger children do this sort of thing naturally, unintentionally, and refreshingly.

*Other Ways of Relaxing.* In contrast to the technique described above, which has a cookbook flavor, we all discover and enjoy ways of relaxation that seem particularly and organically ours. Among children, these (and others) are common:

- Self-massage and self-grooming: rubbing, especially feet; slow hair-brushing; picking the lint out of toes and other crevices.
- Rocking in a chair or on a horsey.
- Listening to music or a story; nonattentive television-watching, with the sound and picture only serving to blot out more immediate sensory impressions, memories, and plans.

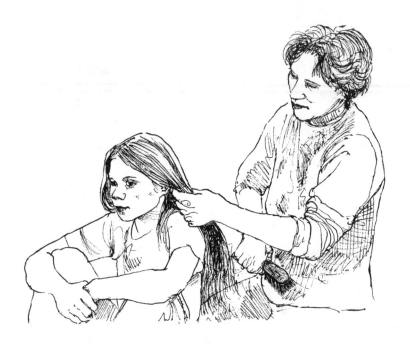

Relaxation: hairbrushing and reverie

- Drinking — especially something warm, like herbal tea, cocoa, or milk — alone in a comfortable chair.
- Taking a long shower or bath, especially with fragrant herbs in the water.
- Walking slowly — wandering, really — with little attention to direction and distance.
- Squatting to watch a hill of ants, the progress of a caterpillar, or the wavings of a crab.

Each of these is a variant of the relaxation response, involving comfort, minimal exertion, letting go of the world around us, and some repetitive or relatively content-less stimulus.

*Centering I.* There is a more complex and self-conscious technique that some very small children can learn with verbal and modeling instruction from adults or older children. It involves an awareness of one's own breathing and a sense of centering one's energy source.

Breathing is an activity that can either be entirely automatic or entirely voluntary. Breathing is done very differently when we are relaxed than when we are in a stress response. When we intentionally breathe in a relaxed manner we more easily bring on the other bodily and mental aspects of thorough relaxation.

Breathing in the stress response is speeded and focused in the chest, geared for the rapid exchange of oxygen and waste gases as needed in maximum exertion. Breathing in the relaxation response is slow and focused in the abdomen. One begins relaxed breathing by inhaling deeply, expiring slowly and fully, and waiting for the next breath to start itself (it always does!). Lying flat on the floor, on one's back and in a comfortable position, is a good way to allow deep breaths to expand one's abdomen. You and your child can both place a hand on the child's abdomen, to feel the rhythmic rise and fall. Children usually can learn to be aware of abdominal breathing more easily than adults. When the easy in and out, rise and fall are established, one can imagine one's breathing in to extend all the way to a tense shoulder, or to a hand or foot. Or one can imagine breathing *out* through an arm or leg, caressing the limb with gentle breath.

This imaginary placing of the breath from the center — the belly — to every part of the body has the effect of focusing attention on parts of the body that are tense or tight, and bringing a soft limpness that is the essence of relaxation. The young child's easy imagination about bodily processes finds delight in this airy game. I have overheard two preschool children, one learning from the other, utterly certain that the breath is entering and leaving toes, elbows, and fingertips.

*Centering II.* A technique that is more complex conceptually, and therefore more easily understood by children of eight or older, involves thinking about and feeling an internal focus of energy, another form of centering. One begins, again, by lying flat on one's back and imagines the center of one's body. The actual center of gravity in the belly, just below the

belly button for adults and just above for children, feels organically right to most of us and relates to a favorite landmark of
children. Imagining a glow, a fire, the source of one's energy
and power, a solid center of weight originating in that place,
one can then send that glow or weight to other parts of the
body to soften them and make them loose and heavy.

Because this form of centering/relaxation is related to a
centering exercise of exertion, it reminds us that relaxation
and exertion are related and connected. The warm, heavy glow
that seeps and creeps out to ease tense and tired muscles is
the same glow that we pull together, coiled and elastic, for
smooth and graceful action. One of my children, at 9 — having
just learned the technique of centering that glow of energy —
got up after a few minutes of relaxing with me and said, "I feel
as if I could do anything — swim the butterfly, ride my bike
around all sorts of corners and circles, jump up to the sky —
with no effort at all."

*Relaxing with Your Child.* Finally, there are ways of bringing about relaxation that involve two. Mothers know them and
children seek them. Lap-sitting, rocking, singing, or humming
or saying the child's name over and over, caressing, rubbing,
and grooming — all induce the relaxation response in mother
and child alike.

Hair-brushing — not the hurried, sometimes hurtful
freeing of snarls for neatness but the gentle caress of a soft
brush and a steady hand (whether or not the snarls are freed)
— is a favorite excuse for slowing down, body contact, repetitive movement, and a sanctuary of shared peace. So is a back
rub. Sometimes it is impromptu, hands up under the shirt.
Sometimes it is a more formal event, with oil or cream and a
darkened room, massaging not only the back but arms, legs,
head, everywhere. Some children, like some adults, are especially relaxed by a foot massage.

A massage is a sustained sensory experience. It is important not to allow your hands to lose contact with the skin.
There is also verbal massage, the simultaneous repetition of a
song or nonsense phrases, or soothing speech that points
awareness to the relaxation itself ("make your arms limp, feel

how heavy they are, you are becoming loose, I can feel you
getting softer and softer, you are so heavy that you will sink
into this nice, soft bed, you feel as soft as silk, all your energy
is flowing gently, gently"). As always, in relaxation, this focus
on inner states brings a retreat from external demands and a
refreshing of spirit and mind as well as body.

It is also reassuring for a tense, distraught child, or simply
a tired child, or a child who needs sleep and cannot loosen
the energies of active striving, to know that someone can soften
that tension and make her/him feel good and whole again.
Many mothers say that a back and head massage is the best
remedy for a colicky infant, or an older baby who has difficulty
falling asleep.


## Exercise

It is not difficult to look around us and understand why, as
adults, we have lost the joy of movement that all children have.
Partly it is our cultural press for saving and using time pro-
ductively — a compulsion centered in our homes and schools
when we are small and suiting the demands of our paid work
when we are older. We are made to feel guilty about taking
time for ourselves. We have lost, through disuse, the sense of
pleasure in physical activity. And we don't know what kind of
activities we might like to do.

Emphasis on competitive sports (another big business) has
encouraged us to believe that exercise is limited to team sports
or sports that require elaborate and expensive equipment and
facilities. For years my own children, who range over 16 years
in age, have held "floating" ball games in the front yard, con-
stituted according to whatever kind of ball is available and
how many children, of whatever ages and capacities, are par-
ticipants. The purpose of their games is social pleasure, inventive delight, and the sheer press of energy to be expended in
wild and fierce abandon.

There is accumulating research evidence about the health
benefits of regular, hard exercise. We know that obesity,
asthma, and other chronic respiratory difficulties, the tendency

to varicose veins and blood clots in the veins, and the narrow-ing of the arteries of the heart muscle that precedes heart attacks, all improve with a regular schedule of vigorous exer-cise. It seems likely that these problems of dis-ease can also be prevented, to some extent. All of them are a part of the natural aging process that begins before we are 10 years old. If exercise becomes a central focus in our lives, we can strive for the promotion of health and the prevention of dis-ease.

Exercise demands deep breathing, which most of us do not use when we move ourselves gently. Deep breathing as we exert ourselves tones the respiratory system and cleanses the blood of wastes by a full exchange of respiratory gases. Our veins get more and more flabby as we grow older, but muscular exertion both increases the rate of blood flow and keeps the blood moving in veins by the squeezing action of tensed mus-cles. Hearts pump more vigorously during exercise, and the heart itself demands and secures an ample supply of the nu-trients of the blood. As for obesity, the expenditure of energy in exercise is rarely matched by an increase in appetite. While weight loss does require a reduction in intake of calories, ex-ercise helps to gather and tone up flesh on the frame. It is also possible that many of the health hazards associated with being overweight are due to a lack of muscular exertion as much as they are due to the extra bodily work imposed by heaviness.

In addition to these relationships between exercise and the prevention of dis-ease, there are other benefits of exercise related to the promotion of health. Exercise increases muscular strength and physical beauty through the firmness of active muscles. Exercise brings physical grace and agility. Exercise promotes endurance. We go through many of our daily activ-ities with more ease and enjoyment when our muscles are capable and practiced. When we need to make an extraordinary effort, whether for pleasure or achievement or to escape or confront danger, a body that is tuned and toned by exercise is there with reserves. Finally, many kinds of exercise constitute opportunities for relaxation of the mind and spirit.

Children in our culture do exercise. But they may learn as they grow that such play is only for small children; they are taught that they should want to participate only in formal, organized activities at school and in recreation centers. Unless we make some effort to inform them to the contrary they are in danger of losing their own self-initiated pleasure in wild and exhausting activity and to learn simultaneously a disdain for any form of exercise, organized or spontaneous. Alternatively they may learn that exercise means competition to win, or the purchase and use of elaborate equipment, or the following of rules dictated by an authority, a rulebook, or a leader.

As adults we may find it difficult to get back to any enjoyment in exercise. As parents we may be fortunate enough to relearn how to exert our own bodies as we struggle to help our children retain their natural enjoyment of exericse.

*Transportation exercises.* The easiest and least self-conscious forms of exercise are those associated with transportation. Walking, running, and bicycling to and from school or work or the corner grocery store are kinds of whole-body exercise that are available to all of us, excepting perhaps those who live in the suburbs or distant rural areas and who have no place that they can reach except by car or bus.

*Game exercises.* Other kinds of exercise that use the whole-body musculature and can be graded from easy exertion to all-out effort are swimming, games of running-with-a-ball (like basketball), Frisbee games, ice-skating, and cross-country skiing. They can be done alone or with others, are not competitive unless we choose to make them so, and require relatively simple and easy-to-find facilities and equipment. Unlike transportation exercise they do require that time be set aside just for the exercise. Children easily reserve this sort of time and call it play. Mothers who play with their children in these informal games find their own exercise and inform their children that adults also need to take time to play.

*Calisthenics.* These exercises for specific muscle groups are delightful for children to do with parents. In urban neighborhoods where it is not safe to be outside at night and where there are few available facilities for simple sports, calisthenics may be the best choice for mothers and children who want to

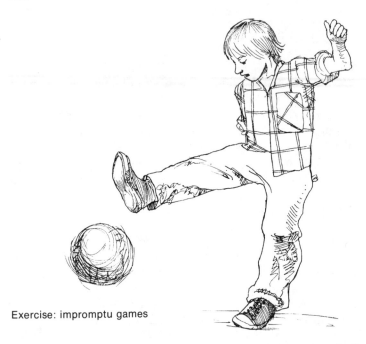

Exercise: impromptu games

exercise together. Calisthenics can be very formal and disci-
plined or can be as informal as loose and energetic dancing to
music.

Easy and comfortable clothing, or no clothing at all, is
essential for strenuous exercise. Ten minutes a day of vigorous
exercise is sufficient for an adult to keep in shape. Children,
of course, will if allowed take much more time for strenuous
exercise. Before mid-childhood children rarely need to be encouraged to run about. What we hope is to stem the cultural
influence that begins to discourage their natural urge for vigorous exercise as they approach adolescence.

The principle of centering, that concentration on the
source of one's energy that is useful in relaxation, is equally
useful as an adjunct to graceful exertion. It is formally a part
of yoga and Samurai training, for instance. Its principle virtue
in exercise, I believe, is to help us become aware of our movements and the connection between mind, body, and spirit in
the process of exercise.

# CHAPTER 7

# Dealing with Medical Professionals

This book argues that mothers can be responsible and competent in giving home health care for their children. This is not the same as arguing that professional care should be avoided. It is true that professional medical care is, for the most part, very expensive, and that it is not equitably available to all. It is also true that professional medical care is geared to taking risks — of harmful effects — in order to save patients from the unhappy consequences of disability, dysfunction, distress, disfigurement, or even death. Doctors and nurses are best at coping with such medical problems as severe burns, broken bones, malignant cancers, congenital malformations that prevent a normal life, and life-threatening birth situations. In these and similar instances the probability of a bad outcome for the patient, were no medical care provided, is so great that doctors can afford to take risks, knowing these risks are *usually* less bad than what the results would be if they did nothing.

For instance, I know a young boy whose right arm has been amputated below the elbow. This amputation occurred when he was ten days old, a prematurely born infant, and had a severe, life-threatening infection. He was so sick that he stopped breathing; in order to get him breathing again while the infection was being treated, the doctors inserted a number of tubes and other devices into him while using a respirator, a machine that breathes for a patient. A clot formed in a tube going into his right arm; the blood supply could not pass into his right hand; the hand and wrist became gangrenous from lack of blood to the tissue, and the amputation had to be performed. He thus lost part of his arm as a direct consequence of the medical care he received.

I know the doctors and nurses who cared for this baby. They were very personally concerned about the loss of his arm. They agonized over whether this amputation could have been prevented; they wondered whether they could have cared for him differently. But the fact is that the treatments they were giving him were inherently dangerous. Before he was well, there were other harmful effects of the treatments. For instance, at one point his kidneys nearly stopped functioning, a known and potentially life-threatening complication of one of the drugs that was used to treat his infection.

In this case, as in so many of the instances when doctors, nurses, and technicians of various sorts do heroic medicine, the alternatives — almost certain death, or almost certain severe mental retardation from an infection that was invading the baby's brain — were worse, to most people's way of thinking, than the side-effect risks of the dangerous treatments. It is important to remember that this is the sort of instance in which our medical-care system works best. This brings about an attitude amongst medical-care workers about risk-taking and their capability for doing harm in the course of trying to do good.

This chapter focuses on two goals. Informed mothers must learn *reasonable expectations* for professional medical care for children. It is hazardous for our children when we expect too much — too much caring, too much prudence, too much restraint, too much wisdom — from those who provide professional medical care. The second goal of this chapter is to assist mothers in becoming *as wise, canny, and self-confident* as possible in the use of the services of medical experts.

As suggested before, most doctors, nurses, technicians, and medical administrators are persons who do care about their patients, care that they do not do harm, care that they mostly do good. Especially — since we *all* care primarily about our-selves — they are concerned about their professional reputa-tions: they want to be known for doing their jobs well. We should not sneer or be unduly cynical about this, for these concerns work to our benefit most of the time.

The *individuals* who work as professional medical experts are neither malevolent nor diabolical. It is the *system* of or-ganized professional medical care that sometimes seems malev-olent and diabolical when it appears to promise us good and then hurts us. We play into this system when we take on the role of naive, trusting, and uninformed patient. We must be very thoughtful about what we ask medical professionals to do for our children. We must understand what we can do, what we can do better than they, what they can do, what they can do better than we, and what risks there are for harm on either side of this equation.

## The Kinds of Help Available from Medical Professionals

*Information and skills.* Doctors, nurses, and technicians have all been through more or less lengthy and complex courses of education and training. They have been taught many facts about disease and disability; some general principles about illness, injury, and healing; and some limited techniques of how to teach others what they know. They have all been told that continuing education is their responsibility, that med-ical information is changing very rapidly — both expanding and being modified — and that they must keep up in their knowledge. They are repositories of medical information. Mothers need access to this information in giving care to their children and in learning how to make judgments about profes-sional medical care. Much of this information is available to parents, as it is to professionals, in libraries. Medical and tech-nical journals, for instance, and medical textbooks are easily accessible and are understandable. A good teacher, however, is often more helpful that a good book. The potential for med-ical professionals to become useful, to-the-point, and inform-ative teachers is very great.

Medical and technical professionals have also been taught numerous skills as part of health assessment and healing assistance. It is more difficult to read a book or a journal and learn a skill than it is to be taught that skill. It is easier to learn how to take the rectal temperature of a baby by being shown by a teacher than by reading about it in a book.

*Diagnostic equipment.* Hospitals and clinics have specialized diagnostic equipment. Sometimes, as with the determination of the hematocrit (see section on ●Hematocrit), the machinery and the process are so simple that anyone could use them; if the purchase price and maintenance costs are not excessive, such equipment could be used by lay groups. In other cases, diagnostic techniques require complex skills. For example, a diagnostic liver biopsy involves sticking a long fine needle through the skin directly into the liver, to pull out a slim core of liver tissue so that the liver cells can be examined under the microscope. Sometimes the interpretation of a diagnostic test requires fine judgment based on lengthy experience. For example, in some blood diseases (such as leukemia or mononucleosis) the blood cells drawn from a vein must be stained and looked at through the microscope for minute changes in size, shape, or color. Some diagnostic equipment is extraordinarily expensive to purchase, intricate to operate, and/or difficult to maintain. For example, the technique of sound scanning, bouncing sound waves off internal structures to identify masses such as tumors and pockets of bleeding, uses machinery that is maintained by engineers. In instances of severe or risky disease, we need to seek the assistance of those who operate such equipment in order to make decisions about appropriate treatments.

*Treatment equipment.* Similarly, hospitals and clinics have treatment equipment that cannot be replicated at home or in simple neighborhood centers. The techniques of surgery are an example. Surgeons can remove parts or masses that cause or result from disease, repair structures to improve their function, or make changes that correct distress or disfigurement. Safe and effective surgery now depends not only on the surgeons' and nurses' clinical skills but also on complex and expensive machinery. Similarly, severe breathing disorders are now treated with elaborate machinery and the backup of lab oratory equipment that determines the composition of the gases dissolved in the blood.

*Signing documents.* Legal requirements now dictate that only physicians (or, in some cases, nurses) can complete and sign certain documents. Among these are prescriptions for restricted drugs; recommendations for special programs in schools; vouchers for government payments in cases of disability; supplies of some drugs, and the like.

## Affecting the behavior of medical experts

When seeking assistance, with regard to children's health, mothers are the *agents* who deal with the medical-care system. Mothers should also educate and change the behavior of medical professionals by pressing for more appropriate and less potentially harmful care. As agents, mothers should oversee the care received by an individual child in a singular instance of disease.

It is critical, however, to keep these two kinds of influence separate. For the most part, watching over the care of an individual child requires defensive strategies. Because the risk of harm at the hands of experts — either from relative inattention or from an overly aggressive approach — is always present, it is rarely appropriate to attempt to educate and change a part of a massive, complex, and highly interrelated system while your child is under professional care. The only exceptions that I know of involve children with lengthy and complicated illnesses — leukemia and other kinds of malignancies, for instance, or cystic fibrosis and other kinds of lifelong dysfunction — when it is clear that they will be continually under care for a very long time, perhaps for all of their lives. In these cases it may be worthwhile, or even necessary, to attempt to alter the principles and philosophy of the care offered by medical professionals. In other instances of care, it is usually best not to risk the kind of negative reaction that is so often an initial response to demands for change.

Efforts to educate and change, on the other hand, have been a notable consequence of the consumer movement in health. Their success has mostly been in small steps, over long periods of time, but has been remarkable all the same. Note for instance changes in hospital policy with regard to parents' visiting their hospitalized children; changes in childbirth procedures, especially with regard to the allowed presence of a nonprofessional person, kin, or friend, to provide significant support to the birthing mother; and changes in parent participation in the care of premature infants. To bring about these sorts of changes we have taken an offensive stance, knowing that we risked resistance or even anger.

*Watching over your child's medical care.* The three guiding principles here are:

- To understand the motives and intents of those who provide care.
- To encourage professional behavior that helps the child.
- To retain as much control as possible, knowing what one's rights are as the responsible parent.

*The motives and intents* of medical professionals are a complicated mixture of wanting to "do good" and striving to maintain the approval of peers and superiors. These two drives are often in conflict. A nurse — especially one who is also a mother — may, for instance, be willing to work with a hospital policy of unlimited visiting by parents of hospitalized children. She may, on the other hand, know that hospital administrators, doctors, and other nurses have been taught that mothers mostly "interfere" with a child's care and influence the child to act badly. Sometimes this means simply that the child in the presence of her/his mother has enough self-esteem and strength to protest against painful or undignified treatment. Interpreting this as "bad" behavior reflects adults' needs and does not respect the child. Research evidence clearly indicates that children recover from disease faster and with fewer complications when they are accompanied in the hospital by parents and other close kin or friends.

Medical work as it is now structured is very frustrating. Medical experts are taught in their training that their job is to make patients well, to save lives, to perform heroic treatments, and never to do harm. As we have acknowledged, most instances of dis-ease cannot be cured by outside agents but are overcome by the body's own healing potential. Most instances of dis-ease are not life-threatening and are not so disabling or dysfunctional as to warrant, much less require, potentially hazardous treatments. Finally, most of the treatments that are the exclusive province of professional medical experts *do* predictably and frequently cause harm. No wonder medical professionals feel frustrated in their work!

It is important to understand these attitudes, motives, and intents of medical professionals. Focusing on their very human qualities of fallibility, self-interest, and disenchantment with their work, as negative characteristics to be disparaged, in no way safeguards your child-as-patient. Remembering instead their wish/hope to do good, the constraints of their talents, and the structure of their work can direct a mother's supervision of medical care for her child that enlists the medical professionals' positive motives and intents.

In a similar manner, we can most effectively *encourage helpful professional behavior* by rewarding medical professionals when they do well. It is easy to grumble about deficiencies, but more difficult to remember to praise for little courtesies. If we receive a pleasant physical space, gentle voices, prompt attention, and full explanation of procedures in a visit to a clinic, we help a child to better professional care by commenting on and praising those things.

This means playing a role as mother-of-the-patient. No one would argue that these relationships *should be* so structured. But they are this way by tradition and by habit. Trying to change them while your child is a patient only puts your child in jeopardy. Playing into them — knowing full well what you are doing — need not be personally demeaning and gives a solid base to your expectations of reasonable consideration for your child's welfare.

Retaining control of your child's care — the third principle — can then be more easily undertaken. Above all, medical professionals believe that they have the responsibility and right to be absolutely and finally in control of every patient-care situation — this despite much recent discussion of the rights of patients. The medical expert's exercise of control comes both from his/her understanding of legal liability (coupled with the knowledge of the risks-for-harm inherent in medical methods) and from the expectation of deference. The control of others is thus professionally justified (as safe practice) and personally justified (as a right). In the long run, retaining as much control as possible over your child's care is far more important for the child than the little games of intentional deference.

A mother's control of her child's care is even more difficult for medical professionals to accept with equanimity than is an adult patient's control of his or her own care. Professional medical experts are often taught, sometimes directly but more often in subtle ways, that mothers are likely to be foolish, uninformed, have difficult relationships with their children, and may be directly responsible for their children's disease. Some of them even see themselves as rescuers of children from parental neglect or ignorance in situations where this is not in fact the case.

However, a mother who is also well-informed about child health, and who respects her own understanding of her own child, has a very good chance of remaining clear-headed about the important decisions that must be made about her child's care.

We have a right to choose which doctor, which clinic, which hospital will care for a child. We have a right to be fully informed about the diagnosis and the reasons why that diagnosis is being entertained. We have a right to know, in advance, what treatments are contemplated, how they are expected to be helpful, and how they might be harmful. We have a right to stay with a child in most medical situations — the most notable exceptions being situations in which the doctor or nurse would be made nervous, and thus endanger the child, by the presence of an observer. We have a right to be informed of new information — laboratory tests, nurses' observations, the observations of repeated physical examination — as the treatments proceed. We have a right to go above the treating physician if we are not being fully informed of the progress of the child in combating her/his disease. ("Above," in a clinic or hospital situation, generally means the administrator, who cares very much about legal liability and public relations.) And we have a right to remove a child from care when we feel that that care may be unduly hazardous or that we are not fully informed of all matters pertaining to the child's welfare.

Precisely because we mothers do care so much for our children, we are inclined to back away when any professional expert seems to tell us that he or she knows more about a child's welfare than we do. While in certain highly risky decision situations the objectivity (lack of direct involvement) of the professional may lend a degree of simplicity to necessary decisions, we must always remember that the professional neither knows the child as well as her/his mother nor cares as much about the outcome for the child. In the end, no one else has the same investment in the child's welfare as the child's mother.

- Choosing a doctor. Several kinds of doctors are qualified to give medical care to children. Pediatricians are specially trained in the diseases of childhood, from the newborn period until adolescence, or in some cases until age eighteen. A family practitioner, a new and more currently trained version of the general practitioner, is also competent in the care of children. While family practitioners often refer to pediatricians in instances of rare or complicated diseases of children, they have the advantage in being able to give care to a child's entire family, and thus the possibility of understanding the impact of an illness

on the dynamics of a household. Internists — specialists
in adult medicine — are sometimes willing to take care of
children past the years of infancy. Some general practitioners remain up-to-date in their medical information and
hold an old-fashioned idea of service to their patients, a
practice that is more rare amongst recently trained
physicians.

Board certification, the passing of written and oral
examinations in a field of specialization, is one mark of an
especially well-qualified physician. Board-certified physicians are not necessarily decent and kindly, nor do they
necessarily remain current in their medical knowledge
*after* they have passed their boards. On the other hand,
some very expert doctors never bother to acquire that extra
certificate of excellence. One can find out whether a doctor
is board-certified by examining the documents hung in her
or his office, or by asking the physician or a nurse, or by
calling the local medical society.

While local medical agencies (the state licensing
board, the physician's medical society, or a smaller —
usually a county — branch of the latter) are generally
recommended as referral sources for physicians, in fact
those offices only weed out doctors who are not licensed
or who have not paid their yearly membership fees. One
gets no recommendation for excellence, either attitudinal
or technical. A much better way of locating a doctor for
one's child is to ask one's friends, inquiring especially
about the doctor's willingness to teach and to answer questions, about the availability of the doctor and the nurse
who works for him or her, and about the personal relationship between your friend and her child, and the doctor. Remember that although many people are very cynical
about medical care in general, most say they are satisfied
with their own physicians.

Doctors work in private practice (administering their
own offices as small businesses), in clinics (as joint owners
with other doctors, or on salary with policy determined in

part by a business administrator), or as salaried staff members in a hospital. Nurses work as salaried employees of doctors, clinics, or hospitals; in any case, nurses work under the medical direction of doctors and sometimes under the nonmedical direction of business administrators. Only recently, and still rarely, do nurses work in a self-directed setting in the private practice of nursing. Technicians — laboratory experts, physical therapists, respiratory therapists, and the like — work, like nurses, under the dual direction of doctors and business administrators. Nurse practitioners, physicians' assistants, and pediatric associates are trained to a level between that of nurses and doctors, functioning in some ways like general practitioners of many years ago. Often they are invaluable resources for mothers because many are devoted to health care (preventive care) rather than just medical care (reparative care) and are intent upon teaching patients what they know. They, too, must, by state law, work under the direction of a physician.

It should be clear that attitudes, competence, and policy are set by doctors themselves. For this reason choosing a doctor for your child is central to the kind of care that your child will receive.

Before visiting a doctor, one should ask over the telephone about short-notice appointment availability. It is less than helpful to visit a physician regularly for checkups only to find that it is impossible to be seen by the doctor when the child is ill. One should, of course, ask about fees. In addition, one should ask about the usual waiting time for an appointment, whether siblings are welcome in the office (in emergency situations when you are unable to find child care), and what hospitals the doctor uses for in-patient care. One should inquire of the hospital what visiting rights are accorded the parents of hospitalized children (unlimited visiting should be expected) and whether the hospital bill must be paid in full before the child is discharged from the hospital. An unwillingness to answer any of these questions is a warning sign; one should look further.

It is, of course, true that in many small-town and rural areas parents have little choice in these matters: there is only one doctor, only one hospital. But in cities there are usually choices to be made, and even in less populous areas it is sometimes reasonable to travel some distance to get better care. In any case, even when no choice is possible, this information is critical to your behavior as a well-informed and thoughtful parent.

- Visiting a doctor. When visiting a doctor, for the first or any later visit, it is always good to ask a friend to accompany you. This rule applies nearly as properly when your child is the patient as when you are the patient, for as the child's mother you are the agent of her/his care and thus subject to the same responsibilities and stresses as an adult patient. The power relationship between doctor and mother is such that it is difficult to remember the questions you wanted to ask, to press for informative and comprehensible answers, and to judge the attitudinal atmosphere of the care given. A friend, not directly involved in the interaction, can give very direct assistance in reality testing: was that nurse really abrupt and cranky with the child, did the doctor really brush aside most of your questions as not worth answering, was the visit as rushed as it seemed to you? Again, if your friend is excluded from the examining or consulting room when you politely request that the friend be allowed to accompany you and your child, that is a warning sign.

However well informed you are about your child and the present status of her/his health, it is good to remember that the doctor will expect you to know the answers to certain questions (birthweight, dates of prior immunizations, ages at which certain developmental milestones like sitting, two-word sentences, and walking were attained) but not much else. Never say to a doctor (until you know him or her well), "I always thought" or "I heard" any so-called *medical* fact. Your information and your questions will be much better respected if you say, "The last doctor we went to told me," or "My father (or uncle), who is a doctor, told me."

You will want your first child to visit a medical professional at regular intervals for a health review. If you have several children and have learned from medical professionals about what happens at each health visit, you may feel that you can carry out the health review yourself. However, you may still wish to consult with a professional about specific questions that have arisen in your own health assessment of the child.

The appropriate intervals for these health visits are more frequent when your child is very young and changing rapidly. Here is a suggested schedule for health visits with a doctor, nurse-practitioner, or physician's assistant:

| at age | 1 month | 9 months | 2 years |
|---|---|---|---|
| | 2 months | 12 months | 2½ years |
| | 4 months | 15 months | 3 years |
| | 6 months | 18 months | |

and yearly thereafter.

At every visit your child should have a complete physical examination, unclothed. The professional should do all the parts of the physical examination outlined in Chapter 3 of this book. In addition, there should be a careful examination of the child's heart, and of all the reflexes and other aspects of the function of the nervous system. You should be asked about your family's history of diseases. You should discuss your child's diet and nutrition, exercise activities and coordination, vision and hearing, sleep, school participation, and relationships with family members and friends. You and your child should have a chance to ask questions about health.

Immunizations and special tests should be done at regular intervals.

*Recommended Schedule of Immunizations*

| AGE | VACCINES |
| --- | --- |
| 2 mos. | DTP (diphtheria, tetanus, pertussis [whooping cough]), TOPV (triple oral polio vaccine) |
| 4 mos. | DTP, TOPV |
| 6 mos. | DTP, TOPV |
| 15 mos. | MMR (measles, mumps, rubella) |
| 18 mos. | DTP, TOPV |
| 4–6 yrs. | DTP, TOPV |
| 14–16 yrs. | TD (tetanus and diphtheria [preparation for adults]) — every ten years |

Special tests should include:

TB test — at 9 months and yearly thereafter.

Sickle-cell test — once only, if you want it done, sometime after 12 months.

Vision test — after the age of 3½ years, there should be a screening exam of the child's vision. For this exam, there are wall charts with pictures of simple objects that the child can recognize and name; there is also the "E-chart," for which the child can indicate the direction of the letter E by holding his fingers pointed in the appropriate direction. (There are training cards that you can take home and use to teach the child how to play this game — some three-year-olds are not able to perform in a visual-acuity exam on the first try.) Vision in both eyes of less than 20/50 is reason for a referral to an ophthalmologist. If vision in one eye differs from that of the other eye by as much as twenty feet (for instance, if one eye gains a score of 20/20 and the other eye gains a score of 20/40), this suggests that the eye with the poorer vision might be a "lazy eye" and the child's vision should be checked by an ophthalmologist.

Lead test — at 12 months, or soon after the child gets around well enough to explore the house. Every 6 months thereafter until age 3, then every year until age 6.

Urinalysis — every year after the child is able to give a urine specimen.

Hemoglobin or hematocrit — every year.

Hearing test (audiometry), if needed.

G6PD. Any child with Mediterranean kin or with dark skin should be tested for a condition called G6PD deficiency. This blood test is usually included in the screening test for sickle-cell disease and trait. The deficiency is the result of the body's inability to produce an enzyme, glucose-6-phosphate dehydrogenase. The significance of this individuality of metabolism is that such persons cannot safely use a variety of drugs, including sulfa drugs and aspirin, without a risk of damage to their red blood cells, resulting in anemia, jaundice, and other potentially serious problems. About 5 percent of the U.S. population has this metabolic deficiency.

Of course, these or other special tests might also be done at other times if there is a particular reason for doing them.

Nurses and social workers are very well trained to work with doctors. They know how to present information to a doctor, describing in accurate detail the patient's entire situation but leaving to the doctor the pronouncement of the diagnosis. It is far more useful for the child if you learn to act like a nurse, describing what you know by your eyes and ears and hands, than to try to beat the doctor to a diagnostic label. On the one hand, if you say, "I think my child has a strep throat," it is possible that your child might get a quick injection of penicillin, when a careful examination and a throat culture would have been more appropriate. On the other hand, I know of one case where that same diagnostic opener led to such irritation in the doctor that no throat culture was done — the doctor unconsciously showing the mother that only *he* could make a diagnosis. It is far more useful for all if you begin by saying, "Susie has had a fever of 101 to 103 degrees for the last 24 hours; she says it hurts when she swallows, and there are some lumps under her jawbone that she says are painful to push at; she has not eaten well for the last day; and her best friend at school had a throat culture two days ago that was reported to show strep."

Of course, it is better to avoid the temptation to react to real or presumed insults in the midst of a care situation. I think that doctors' (and sometimes nurses') irritability about "uppity" mothers is at least partly a reaction to the women's movement and to the consumer movement in health matters. If your child is demeaned and you do not need to return to that doctor, you can of course simply cut the visit short. Otherwise, you can deal with the insult after your child is no longer in care.

You are entitled to answers to all questions about the results of the examination, about the doctor's diagnoses and the reasons for these conclusions, about the exact treatments to be recommended, their effects and their possible side effects. You are entitled to be taught any skill that you might use at home. If you are told that the doctor or other staff are too busy to teach you, you are entitled to ask when you may come back to the office for that teaching. No visit to a doctor, except in very special circumstances, should involve less than fifteen minutes of direct contact with professional staff, or less than ten minutes of the doctor's time, if you choose to use that time. No visit should leave you with unanswered questions and no offer of follow-up time when your questions will be answered. Don't forget to ask your children, when they are old enough, what questions they want to ask and have answered.

Any visit for medical care in which a problem has been found will have some follow-up, either to discover how the condition is progressing or to learn when prescribed treatments have been helpful. Ask when that follow-up is to be scheduled; who is available to you by telephone and when; how you are to know whether the condition is getting better or worse; and what danger signs or side effects you are to watch for.

Before any drastic measures are taken with your child,

such as surgery, a dangerous medicine, or restriction from normal activities, it is good to get a second opinion, either from another doctor at a similar level of specialization as the first doctor or from a more specialized doctor. That is, if a pediatrician has recommended surgery one may get a second opinion from another pediatrician, from a general surgeon, or from a pediatric surgeon. If you have health insurance, you should check your policy or ask your insurance agent whether this second-opinion visit will be paid for by your insurance. If you get two conflicting opinions, you must then decide which of the two seems most reasonable to you, or else seek still another opinion. It is important (if possible) to get a second opinion from a doctor who is not an acquaintance of the first doctor.

Until you are very confident of the care your child gets from doctors, nurses, and technicians, stay with your child at all times. Except in very rare and unusual situations, there is no procedure that cannot be performed with a parent present. If you feel faint at the sight of needles or blood, perhaps your friend can stay with the child until you overcome your faintness. Not only will your child be comforted by your presence — and maybe feel able to protest treatment that is thoughtless or painful — but also you cannot know what is done or said to your child unless you are present.

Most doctors, and the staffs of clinics and hospitals, are continually nervous that bills for services given will not be paid. You are never obliged to pay for care before it is given, or on that same day. But it is courteous and safeguarding for the future care you and your child will get to acknowledge bills when they are received and to pay something, even a small amount, with an explanation of your plans for paying the balance. Doctors' offices, clinics, and hospitals in this country, at this time, must be run as businesses; you or your child may be ill-treated in the future if you ignore your bills. On the other hand, you are quite in order if you pay some small amount every month. You should also know that any clinic or hospital that has used federal funds for its building is obliged to provide some care at no charge. Most clinics and hospitals have a sliding scale of fees, assigned according to family income. And all states have funds for medical assistance to families below certain income levels. Hospitals and clinics have personnel in their business or social-service offices to help families apply for these entitlements.

Finally, if you are partially satisfied with the care your child has received and partially dissatisfied, do not give up too quickly. Like all human relationships, doctor-patient and nurse-patient connections require repeated contact to develop. Make separate visits with each of your children, instead of bringing all of them at one time. Make telephone calls. Initial attitudes of disinterest and coldness often vanish after you and the medical staff come to know each other. You *can* train your doctor!

## How to Educate and Change Medical Professionals

The consumer movement of recent years has taught us a great deal about the power of the purchaser. No matter how frustrating and inappropriate it may seem to think of medical care as a commodity that is bought and sold, we can use that fact as the basis of a community effort to improve the medical care available to our children.

The first key to success lies in the word community. This is no place for a one-person campaign, no matter how courageous. As long as you have children who may need medical care, you jeopardize their well-being by seeming to be an outspoken leader in a movement for change. By acting in concert with other mothers you blur your individual identity and thus protect your children.

If you are not satisfied with the care you child is receiving you can boycott that doctor, either going elsewhere for care or working to bring another doctor to your community. More directly, you can write a letter to the doctor (or clinic, or hospital) indicating the reasons for your dissatisfaction and asking for a meeting to discuss problems.

In addition to direct approaches to the doctor, there are other avenues of approach. The nurse or nurses who work with that doctor may also be mothers. Unless their professionalism is absolutely separated from their motherhood, they may be persuaded to understand the reasons for your dissatisfaction. If they are competent and valued employees, they may be able to advise the doctor to change office policy. In clinics and hospitals there are business administrators who are very concerned with public image and public relations. Although doctors greatly dislike having medical policy dictated by nonmedical administrators, sometimes they have no choice.

Find out where monies come from for doctors' salaries. If a clinic or hospital is funded by state or federal funds, such as from the Department of Health, Education and Welfare, take your complaints directly to the local office that administers these funds. In states where Blue Cross/Blue Shield or some other health-insurance company is very active, you may have some success in going directly to the insurance company and applying pressure in that way. Similarly, the offices that administer state medical assistance monies will often be interested in such complaints.

There are other, rather more traditional, methods for relating to those who give unsatisfactory medical care to children. One of these is not to pay bills for care that seems to be careless or attitudinally inappropriate. This is perfectly reasonable if you do not wish to use that source of medical care again. For many, however, there are few or even no alternatives but to work with the only doctor or clinic in your community. While not paying bills on a matter of principle is a powerful weapon, it is also likely to be so alienating to the professionals that it will make future dealings very difficult if not impossible.

Suits for damages fall in the same category. If a child or a family has been hurt by negligent care, one should certainly sue. On the other hand, this is a method of punishment and is not at all likely to change professional behavior for the better. If you wish to or must continue to use the same professional resources, a suit or the threat of a suit will interfere with other methods of inducing change.

If your town has a community or school health committee (usually headed by a doctor or a strong school nurse) you may focus the attention of that committee on your complaints. Lawyers, ministers, other doctors, and prominent businessmen might find your issues of public-relations value and be willing to lend their names if not their voices to your efforts.

Over and above the changing of specific practices and policies, there is the whole matter of the responsiveness of medical professionals to community needs. Are children in your community at risk of lead poisoning? Is your pediatrician vigorously testing children's blood for lead levels, working with the town's lead-inspection office, adding her or his name to lobbying efforts for local ordinances or state laws that are effective in requiring landlords to remove lead paint from dwellings occupied by young children? Has he or she encouraged the formation of a parents' action group and shared recent medical-journal information about the lead-poisoning problem?

How appropriate to health needs is the physical-education program in your local schools? Is your children's doctor actively working with school personnel to consider this and other educational activities directed toward health? What coordination is there between medical care in doctors' offices, clinics, and hospitals and health supervision in the schools on such matters as annual health certificates, surveillance for school-based epidemics of infectious disease, first-aid for injuries, and the like? What are the resources available in school and from professional medical experts for parents to provide sex education for their children?

Do your children know first-aid techniques appropriate to their ordinary activities? What health-related information would parents like to learn? Who are the special-needs children in your community, in your schools? What community-based efforts are being made to understand and help these children and their families?

What are the major nutritional needs of children in your community? How available is nonprocessed food — at what convenience and at what cost? Is there a neighborhood food cooperative for buying fresh produce and other staples? Are families who are entitled to government-based food supplements (such as food stamps and the Women, Infants and Children [WIC] Program) helped to apply for this assistance? Is there a garden cooperative so that community families can share equipment, skills, and energies to provide locally grown produce for their own tables?

In these and other community concerns professional medical experts have some information, some skills that can be directed to matters of interest to community groups. If, as one would hope, the medical professionals live in the neighborhoods in which they work, these concerns are in their own self-interest. Community health advisory groups can direct the attention of medical professionals to these general community concerns. In particular, a mothers' committee can serve as such an advisory group.

## What a Health Committee Could Do

In keeping with the idea that group efforts are more effective than individual efforts, consider the formation of a mothers' health committee in your community. Mothers of children of all ages can be found at school or day-care meetings, at the places where you work, at neighborhood centers or church organizations; their collective experience with the local doctors, clinics, and hospitals will be very great. A group of mothers with similar goals for the good health of their children can become a mothers' health committee and an effective force for change.

In addition to drawing attention to health problems generally present in the community, a mothers' health committee could request or demand the following kinds of cooperation between medical professionals and families:

● The opening of office or clinic records about the care given to each child. Better, copies of these records should be given to parents, to be held in trust until a child is old enough to maintain her/his own health records. It is impractical to expect doctors to hold medical records for individuals; no one has a greater interest in such records than the person who is the subject of the records. Accounts of the historical development of traits of health and dis-ease, of the findings at physical examinations, of diagnoses made, of treatments given, and of the process of healing, are often invaluable in instances of dis-ease in later life.

- The establishment of a clear policy of assistance for home health care, including telephone consultations and home visiting to confirm mothers' observations and techniques of care. One can expect that professional services will incur charges on the basis of time spent and materials used. Home care assistance will not be provided free, but in the long run — as you learn examination and treatment skills — your competence will result in fewer expenses for professional assistance. In my own practice I clearly re-member two groups of mothers with years of mothering behind them. One group had always assumed a passive stance with regard to professional assistance, and chose to belittle or demean what they had learned about child health in the course of long and extensive experience in child-rearing; often their attitude in the clinic was sullen, and I expect that somewhere in their heads they knew how much they really knew. The other group adopted an ag-gressive posture of knowledge and canniness: they knew, and wanted my acknowledgment, that they were experts in managing their children's dis-ease. I believe that the attitudes of the first group arose in large part from their experiences with doctors, nurses, and technicians who had refused to credit the validity of mothers' experience. De-mands for a policy of assistance to home health care should begin with an insistence on the validity of mothers' experience.

- Regularly scheduled meetings between the mothers' health committee and the professional medical experts who serve child health needs in your community. The responsibility for the agenda of these meetings must lie with the mothers' committee. Appropriate topics might include: recently noticed community problems in or barriers to child health; the attitudes of professionals toward lay persons, especially mothers; specific teaching, in lay-comprehensible language, about common child-health problems; requests that professionals identify written resources, in medical textbooks and journals, about particular questions in child health; and discussions of bureaucratic policies (for instance, the policies of your local hospital) with regard to children and their parents.

## Organizations

There are organizations that might take to heart the concerns of parents who provide home health care for their children. Parents are eligible for membership in these organizations and thus can determine the agenda. These organizations include:

- Health systems agencies. Mandated by the federal government, these agencies must be composed of both service providers (doctors, nurses, technicians, administrators, and the like) and consumers. The primary concerns of these agencies are related to the local expenditure of federal health funds, and include health planning, cost control, programs, building, and equipment. The rather homely (but, as we know, very important) issues that concern mothers and children are not so likely to involve expenditures of federal funds. Nonetheless, some HSAs have spoken strongly for more general issues — patients' rights and patients' access to their own records — that affect the care of children.
- Boards of trustees of hospitals. Appointed or nominated by a variety of mechanisms, these boards have some power over the behavior of professionals in the hospital setting (but not outside) and some authority to set or ratify hospital policy. Because the people who have the time to serve on hospital boards are usually past the age of rearing children, the concerns of children usually take a low priority in their deliberations. Again, your presence as a board member might affect those priorities.
- Town boards of health, school boards, and other positions

in local (town, city, or county) government. These offer other outlets to represent the health needs of children and their mothers. They all have some degree of influence over local health matters.

A mothers' health committee might lobby to have one of their members on each of these and similar local health agencies. In this way the best interests of children and their caretakers can be represented.

# CONCLUSION

A major purpose of this book has been to urge mothers to recognize how simple most techniques of medical care for children really are. We have been so conditioned to believe that what doctors and nurses do is complex and complicated, beyond the grasp of layfolk that we have often shied away from hearing about healing at home.

A second major intent has been to clarify the meaning of the threat that if we do not seek professional consultation for every sniffle and hurt, we might risk the well-being of our children. Sometimes ordinary symptoms, like vomiting or headache, have ominous significance. We can learn when those problems should be brought to professional attention, and when we can deal with them ourselves. We all do know — no matter how driven we might feel to seek endless professional advice — that most dis-ease experienced by children can be competently cared for at home. We need guidelines and examples to think through the reasons for seeking professional consultation.

A final hope has been that mothers might regain a sense of competence and good feeling about caring for children, in their illnesses and injuries, at home. The role of women as healers has progressively been denied to us with the rise of the medical professionals as advisers in our everyday lives. I do in fact believe that professional advice should be readily available and respectfully given; I do not think that the welfare of children or the welfare of mothers — the principle caretakers of children — is increased when that advice is conveyed as "Let me take over." If, instead, that advice were given as "Let me teach you," mothers could again appreciate that they are already essential assistants in their children's healing. What we already do well we can learn to do better by appreciating our own potential for competence.

The welfare and well-bring of children is greatly dependent on and responsive to mothers' sense of self-esteem and contentment. To recognize this is not to say that mothers have a duty and obligation to "be happy" for the sake of their children; no burden could be more onerous. But mothers do have a right, for the sake of their children as well as for their own sakes, to remind others of the quality of this connection. When mothering is demeaned or unsupported, children are put at risk. When mothers are personally made to feel incompetent and foolish, their children suffer consequences. If, on the other hand, mothers feel supported in their efforts to care for children, that care can only be better. When we learn skills in home health care, when we understand the process of assisting our children in their own healing, and when we provide thoughtful and competent care in specific instances of dis-ease, our children thrive not only in the process of care but in the reflected light of our own self-esteem.

The examples of care given in this book are meant to illustrate a process. Throughout, you have been urged to ask professionals to teach you, to explain and demonstrate what else you need to know. No home-health encyclopedia can cover every instance in which you will need to help your child heal — human dis-ease too rarely falls into neat patterns, appears in a classical or textbook form, or repeats itself even in the course of rearing several children. For each specific episode of dis-ease in your child or children, there will be information and skill-learning that you can helpfully gain through professional consultation.

The book has focused on relatively simple kinds of disease, of the sort that you will probably care for at home. Professionals sometimes need to be reminded that these kinds of disease are important to the child and to her/his mother, and that they can in fact be helpful not by taking over but by giving consultative advice. In the context of this book, "Ask your doctor" does not mean "Ask him or her to provide heroic care."

Most of us learn a great deal about our own bodies in the course of caring for our children's illnesses and injuries. Most important, perhaps, we learn about the importance of remedies that comfort and that support self-healing. In turn, we can pass what we know along to our children. We can begin again to generate and respect that chain of healing skills and understanding that has traditionally been the province of women and is centered in home, neighborhood, and community. As we teach our children to be skillful and respectful of their own bodies, their own potential for self-healing, and their own competence to assist others in healing, we will widen the healing community to include all who wish to learn to care.

# Selected Bibliography

The following list of books is a sampling of the kinds of printed information useful to mothers who wish to become more competent in and thoughtful about providing health care at home for their children. Most of these books are useful as reference manuals, to be looked at for specific information from time to time; some are informative in a single reading.

These books have been written by experts of many persuasions. Their formal credentials (that is, professional degrees) are indicated only if they are members of the care-giving medical establishment. This limited identification is by no means meant to imply that physicians and nurses are more believable than those without credentials. The books written by non-credentialed people can oftentimes be exceedingly helpful in the home health care of children.

It should be obvious that I do not recommend that a single household buy and own all these and other similar books. A community center or neighborhood group could buy and own some, and share them with its members. Others could be made available in a local library; libraries do respond to the requests of groups of users in the purchase of new books. A mothers' group could request that a clinic, hospital library, or private physician maintain an up-to-date selection of books about child health, and make those books available to parents.

## Attitudes toward health and medical care:

Children's Defense Fund, *EPSDT: Does it Spell Health Care for Poor Children?* Washington Research Project, Inc., 1520 New Hampshire Avenue, N.W., Washington, DC 20036, 1977.

Analysis of the intent and the actual outcome of medical assistance programs for poor children funded by the federal and state governments.

Illich, Ivan, *Medical Nemesis: The Expropriation of Health*, Pantheon, New York, 1976.

A tremendously informative book about the consequences of medical care on the health of individuals in our society, and a thought-provoking discussion about human ills and our attitudes about perfectability.

Schrag, Peter, and Divoky, Diane, *The Myth of the Hyperactive Child and Other Means of Child Control*, Pantheon Books, New York, 1975.

A thorough and sensible discussion of the "medicalization" of a childhood condition that has many social, educational, and philosophic connections. A thought-provoking book that reminds us of the dangers of converting all of the ills of living into conditions with medical explanations and medical treatments.

## Home health care

Alexander, Mary M., R.N., M.S., and Brown, Marie Scott, R.N., Ph.D., *Pediatric Physical Diagnosis for Nurses*, McGraw Hill, New York, 1974.

A very valuable book for mothers. Although not written in strictly lay language, the procedures of the physical examination are explained and discussed thoroughly, and glossaries help clarify the language used.

Barness, Lewis A., M.D., *Manual of Pediatric Physical Diagnosis*, Year Book Medical Publishers, Inc. Chicago, 1972.

Written for medical students, the language of this handbook is not designed for lay readers. Nonetheless, with professional consultation (needed, in any case, for learning the practical procedures of physical examination) the book is very useful for mothers.

The Boston Women's Health Book Collective, *Our Bodies, Our Selves*, Simon and Schuster, New York, 1976.

This invaluable book is a model of how health-related information, of the sort needed by laywomen to make informed decisions about themselves, can be found and shared by persons who are not medical professionals. Its perspectives help mothers to gain control and responsibility for their own health, and thus enable mothers to think more clearly about control and responsibility for the health of their children. It is also an important resource book for adolescent girls.

Brodsky, Greg, *From Eden to Aquarius: The Book of Natural Healing,* Bantam Books, New York, 1974.

Chapters on water treatments, diet, massage, exercise and relaxation, especially from the perspective of Eastern cultures.

Brown, Marie Scott, R.N., Ph.D., and Murphy, Mary Alexander, R.N., M.S., *Ambulatory Pediatrics for Nurses,* McGraw-Hill Book Company, New York, 1975.

Most of the information in this book is directly useful to mothers, although relatively little is said about home treatment of complains and disorders. There is an especially good section on special diagnostic tests, for example of vision, hearing, speech.

*Child Health Record,* The American Academy of Pediatrics, Evanston, Illinois.

One model for a home health record, suggesting some of the categories of information that should be included. Too little space is allotted for recording the history and findings of episodes of illness.

*Common Medical Terminology,* Abbott Laboratories, North Chicago, Ill., 60064.

A handy glossary of medical terms. Available free.

Copans, Stu, and Osgood, David, *The Home Health Handbook,* Stephen Greene Press, Brattleboro, Vt., 1972.

A very practical guide to home health care, mostly for adults.

Cunningham, P. J., *Nursery Nursing,* Faber and Faber, London, 1967.

A book about home nursing procedures, especially for young babies.

Hoole, Axalla J., M.D., Greenberg, Robert A., M.D., Pickard, C. Glenn, Jr., M.D., eds. *Patient Care Guidelines for Family Nurse Practitioners,* Little, Brown, Boston, 1976.

These guidelines are directed to nurse practitioners who take care of families. There is much information directly about infants and children. The book is explicit about when to consult a physician for a child who has various symptoms and signs of disease.

Kloss, Jethro, *Back to Eden,* Lifeline Books, Santa Barbara, CA, 1972.

A compendium of suggestions about healthful eating, the use of water treatments for illness, and herbal remedies. As with all

similar books (including medical textbooks) one needs to consider the arguments given for the use of a remedy or treatment,
balance the risk of harm against the potential benefit, try the
remedy yourself, and then make a decision about using the remedy for your child.

Law, Donald, *A Guide to Alternative Medicine*, Doubleday, New York,
1976.

A brief encyclopedia of theory and technique in alternative medical treatments.

Popenoe, Chris, *Wellness*, Yes! Inc., 1035 31st Street, N.W., Washington, D.C. 20007.

This book is an annotated list of books on various topics in health
and healing, including some traditional and some innovative
approaches that are not part of standard medical care in this
country.

Samuels, Mike, M.D., and Bennett, Hal, *The Well Body Book*, Random
House, New York, 1973.

A manual of home health care for adults.

Samuels, Mike, M.D., and Bennett, Hal, *Be Well*, Random House, New
York, 1974.

Some ideas about self healing.

Sobel, David S., and Hornbacher, Faith L., *An Everyday Guide to
Your Health*, Grossman, New York, 1973.

A home health care book, mostly but not exclusively for adults,
oriented to health rather than to illness and injury.

### Remedies

Buchman, Dian Dincin, *The Complete Herbal Guide to Natural Health
and Beauty*, Doubleday, New York, 1973.

General instructions for preparing herbal remedies, and a delightful collection of suggestions for home made substances to rub on
the skin. Sensible discussion of diet as it affects skin and hair. As
enjoyable for adolescents as it is for mothers. There is a helpful
section on adolescent skin troubles.

Buchman, Dian Dincin, *Organic Make-up*, Ace Books, New York,
1975.

Simple recipes for shampoos, soaps, massage oils, and so on,
from natural ingredients. Your children can join you in making
these, or make them by themselves.

Catzel, Pincus, *The Paediatric Prescriber*, Blackwell Scientific Publications, London, 1974.

Written for medical professionals, this is a formulary of drugs used for children.

Graedon, Joe, *The People's Pharmacy: A Guide to Prescription Drugs, Home Remedies and Over-the-Counter Medications*, Avon, New York, 1976.

Primarily about adults and written in a rather breezy style, this book has some information relevant to treating children, such as warnings about drug interactions. Some good tips on home treatment are also given, and there is a useful chart on the costs of brand-name buying.

Grieve, M., *A Modern Herbal*, Dover Publications, New York, 1971.

Careful, comprehensive review of the herbs used in Western diets and as remedies.

Kadans, Joseph, *Encyclopedia of Medicinal Herbs*, Arco Publishing, New York, 1970.

An encyclopedic book about herbs recommended for specific conditions, and the healing properties that have been attributed to specific herbs.

Levy, Juliette de Baïracli, *Nature's Children: A Guide to Organic Foods and Herbal Remedies for Children*, Warner Paperback, New York, 1972.

A book specifically about mothering, this small volume is full of old wisdom.

Levy, Juliette de Baïracli, *Common Herbs for Natural Health*, Schocken Books, New York, 1974.

A compendium of ways of using herbs, methods of preparing them, and their possible effects as remedies, written by a mother.

Long, James W., M.D., *The Essential Guide to Prescription Drugs*, Harper and Row, New York, 1977.

Not about children, but has information about drugs that you might give to a child.

Morton, Julia F., *Folk Remedies of the Low Country*, E. A. Seeman Publishing, Miami, 1974.

A scholarly, regional, herbal encyclopedia, a model of the sort of contemporary and traditional information that we should have available for every local region.

Null, Gary, and Null, Steve, *Herbs for the Seventies*, Dell Books, New York, 1972.

Chapters on some specific herbs, such as licorice, nettle, and alfalfa, that might be used for health.

Parish, Peter, M.D. *The Doctors' and Patients' Handbook of Medicines and Drugs*, Knopf, New York, 1977.

This plain-spoken book is an excellent and comprehensive reference on how substance remedies work, their benefits and hazards, and what precautions should be used in deciding on their use. It is not directly about children, but the information presented is for the most part as applicable to children as to adults. Herbal substances are not discussed.

*Physicians' Desk Reference to Pharmaceutical Specialties and Biologicals* (PDR), Medical Economics Company, Inc., Oradell, N.J., published yearly, and amended quarterly.

This is a standard reference book. It contains brief discussions of all prescription drugs; each discussion is the same as the package insert that you can get from the pharmacist, if you ask, when you buy a prescription. These discussions are now often used as reference standards to "good practice," for instance, in malpractice suits. Included is information on the indications for which the drug should be given and its method of action, the recommended dosage, common side effects, and so on. An invaluable home reference book.

Rau, Henrietta A. Diers, *Healing with Herbs*, Arco Publishing, New York, 1968.

An encyclopedic book about herbs recommended for specific conditions, and the healing properties that have been attributed to specific herbs.

Twitchell, Paul, *Herbs: The Magic Healers*, Illuminated Way Press, P.O. Box 82388, San Diego, CA, 92138.

Interesting discussion of herbs as foods and remedies, based mostly on the traditions of Eastern cultures.

Weiner, Michael A., *Earth Medicine, Earth Foods*, Collier Books, New York, 1972.

Information about plant remedies and natural foods native to North America.

## Illnesses and injuries of childhood

Altshuler, Anne, R.N., M.S., *Books that Help Children Deal with a Hospital Experience*, U.S. Department of Health, Education and

Welfare, Public Health Service, Health Services Administration. Bureau of Community Health Services, 5600 Fishers Lane, Rockville, Maryland, 20852.

An annotated bibliography of books for children. Purchase for 50¢ from the Superintendent of Documents, U.S. Government Printing Office, Washington, D.C. 20402.

The Boston Children's Medical Center and Feinbloom, Richard I., M.D. *Child Health Encyclopedia: The Complete Guide for Parents*, Delacorte Press/Seymour Lawrence, Boston, 1975.

A useful sourcebook for mothers, although not focussed on home-based care and therefore often skewed in the kind and detail of information offered. The information here is useful and necessary, but often insufficient to guide home care.

Committee on Hospital Care, *Care of Children in Hospitals*, American Academy of Pediatrics, P.O. Box 1034, Evanston, Illinois, 60204.

Guidelines for professionally thorough and responsible care for hospitalized children.

Committee on Standards of Child Health Care, *Standards of Child Health Care*, The American Academy of Pediatrics, Evanston, Illinois, 60204, 1972.

Although oriented more to medical care than to health, this volume is the official pediatric recommendation for standards in professional supervision of the health of children.

DeAngelis, Catherine, M.D., R.N. *Basic Pediatrics for the Primary Health Care Provider*, Little, Brown, Boston, 1975.

Although this book is not addressed to mothers, it contains a wealth of information about common childhood dis-ease, including information about recommended medical treatment. Not much information is given, however, about home remedies.

Dynski-Klein, Martha, *Color Atlas of Pediatrics*, Year Book Medical Publishers, Inc., Chicago, 1975.

A collection of color photographs of abnormal and unusual conditions of childhood. Most of these are relatively rare, but some of the more common conditions are also included.

Graef, John W., M.D. and Cone, Thomas E., M.D. *Manual of Pediatric Therapeutics*, Little, Brown, Boston, 1974.

A handbook on pediatric diseases and their remedies, written for professionals.

Hendlin, David, *Save Your Child's Life!*, Doubleday and Co., Garden City, New York, 1974.

A short book about accidents, including poisonings, especially those in the home setting. Some first-aid measures are discussed, but most of the accidents discussed require hospital-based treatment. There are good reminders about learning cardio-pulmonary resuscitation (mouth-to-mouth breathing and external heart massage), which everyone should understand and practice at intervals.

Kempe, C. Henry, M.D., Silver, Henry K., M.D., O'Brien, Donough, M.D., *Current Pediatric Diagnosis and Treatment,* Lange Medical Publications, Los Altos, CA, 1978.

A standard pediatric reference book used by professional experts in the medical care of children.

Reece, Robert M., M.D., and Chamberlain, John W., M.D. *Manual of Emergency Pediatrics,* Saunders, Philadelphia, 1974.

Very technical and hospital-oriented. Helpful to mothers as a reference manual for serious, often life-threatening emergency conditions. A few less severe conditions treatable at home are included.

Rudolph, Abraham M., M.D., ed., *Pediatrics,* Appleton, Century, Crofts, New York, 1976.

A standard pediatric reference book used by professional experts in the medical care of children.

Shirkey, Harry C., M.D., ed., *Pediatric Therapy,* Mosby, Saint Louis, 1975.

A standard pediatric reference book used by professional experts in the medical care of children.

Vaughn, Victor C., M.D. ed., *Textbook of Pediatrics,* Saunders, Philadelphia, 1975.

A standard pediatric reference book used by professional experts in the medical care of children.

Waisbren, Burton A., M.D., *Emergency Care,* Drake Publishers, Inc., New York, 1975.

Suggestions for readiness for medical emergencies (a list for a home first-aid kit, checklists for selecting ambulance service, hospital emergency rooms, and the like), combined with brief discussions about common medical problems, emergent and non-emergent, of concern to adults. Some information is relevant to children and health.

## Nutrition

Brewer, Gail S., *What Every Pregnant Woman Should Know: The Truth about Diets and Drugs in Pregnancy*, Random House, New York, 1977.

A valuable book about nutrition for the unborn child. Although many of the practical suggestions assume that mothers have more time and money than many of us do, the book as a whole is very important and useful.

Jacobson, Michael, *Nutrition Scoreboard: Your Guide to Better Eating*, Center for Science in the Public Interest, 1779 Church Street, N.W., Washington DC, 20036, 1973.

Particularly useful for its analysis of the composition of brand-name foods that children ask for and that mothers wonder about the nutritional value of.

Jarvis, D. C., M.D., *Folk Medicine*, Fawcett Crest, Greenwich, Conn., 1958.

Discussions about honey, apple cider, dietary potassium seaweed, and other naturally-occurring healthful foods.

Lansky, Vicki, *Feed Me, I'm Yours*, Meadowbrook Press, 16648 Meadowbrook Lane, Wayzata, Minnesota, 55391, 1974.

This delightful "recipe book for mothers" is a good guide to nutritious and appealing foods, especially for the baby not yet ready to share adult meals.

Lappe, Frances Moore, *Diet for a Small Planet*, Ballantine Books, New York, 1971. (And the companion volume *Recipes for a Small Planet*, Ellen B. Ewald, Ballantine Books, New York, 1975.)

A comprehensive and very readable account of the wastefulness of our habits of intensive meat-eating, and an argument for more thoughtful use of vegetable sources of iron- and protein-containing foods. Every household should be familiar with this book.

Longgood, William, *The Poisons in your Food*, Pyramid Books, New York, 1960.

An early but still-useful book on pollution and processing in the food industry.

Seaman, Barbara S., and Seaman, Gideon S., *Women and the Crisis in Sex Hormones*, Rawson, New York, 1977.

The section on "Menopause: Wholesome Remedies" is an excellent review of the nutritional importance of various foodstuffs, vitamins, and minerals, applicable to children as well as to adult women.

*Sugar and How it Gets That Way,* Talking Food Company, Box 81, Charlestown, MA, 02129, 1977.

One of a series of short pamphlets about some of the foodstuffs that we take for granted.


## Relaxation

Downing, George, *The Massage Book,* Random House, New York, 1972.

A pleasant book about a variety of massage techniques.

Miller, Roberta DeLong, *Psychic Massage,* Harper Colophon Books, New York, 1975.

A book about massage techniques, with a thoughtful discussion of the psychic energies involved in the experience of massage.

Rush, Anne K., *Getting Clear,* Random House, New York, 1973.

Techniques of relaxation, discussed from the perspective of adult women but useful for children as well.


## Exercise

Lettvin, Maggie, *The Beautiful Machine: Your Own Body,* Ballantine Books, New York, 1972.

More on calesthenics, including some slow-starters for the out-of-shape.

Levy, Janine, *The Baby Exercise Book,* Pantheon Books, New York, 1975.

Games to play with babies (0–15 months) that are pleasurable for children and adults and teach a body awareness to both.

Prudden, Suzy, and Sussman, Jeffrey, *Suzy Prudden's Family Fitness Book,* Simon and Schuster, New York, 1975.

Calesthenics for pregnant and postpartum women and for children and adults of all ages.

Taub, Harold J., *Keeping Healthy in a Polluted World,* Penguin Books, New York, 1974.

A review of environmental pollution and its effects on health.

United States Department of Agriculture, Home and Garden Bulletin
    No. 72, *Nutritive Value of Foods*, Superintendent of Documents,
    U.S. Government Printing Office, Washington, D.C. 20402.

United States Department of Agriculture, Agriculture Research Ser-
    vice, Agriculture Handbook No. 8, *Composition of Foods*, Super-
    intendent of Documents, U.S. Government Printing Office, Wash-
    ington D.C. 20402.

Williams, Roger J., *Nutrition Against Disease*, Bantam Books, New
    York, 1971.

    A discussion of the relationships between the foods we eat and
    preventive health care, by a scientist whose perspective on bio-
    chemical individuality is well-known and important.

# INDEX

# THE AUTHOR

Mary Howell, M.D., Ph.D., received her degrees from Radcliffe College and the University of Minnesota. She is former Director of the Family Evaluation Unit at Massachusetts General Hospital and former Associate Dean of the Harvard Medical School.

While at Harvard, she wrote *Helping Ourselves: Families and the Human Network,* published by Beacon Press in 1975, which encourages families to care for themselves without the overdependency on family care experts. This radical philosophy led Dr. Howell and two other women to open a pediatric clinic, The Child Health Station, in York Corner, Maine.

Dr. Howell, mother of six children, currently lives and practices pediatrics in the Greater Boston area.